Recent Praise

I recently had an older client travel for the first time both as a widow (and therefore alone) along with a recent change in her general physical mobility. She was experiencing significant anxiety as she planned for a cross country trip to visit her daughter; in fact she almost didn't go due to her worries. On her return, the report of her challenges, fears and frustrations rang true with the issues presented in this book.

As a physical therapist working primarily with older adults in an out patient and community setting, I am pleased to be able to recommend *Wheeling and Dealing* as a resource to my clients. I feel the book is stated in simple terms and offers good advice. Although much seems obvious to seasoned travelers—the personal stories and down-to-earth advice make it user-friendly. (I know a few able-bodied travelers who could use some guidance such as this!) I appreciate the fact that the authors discussed much about mobility challenges as well as low vision since both are common in the older adult population. Thank you to the authors for seeing the need beyond yourselves and taking the initiative to provide guidance and relevant information for traveling with disability.

—*Kathryn K Brewer, PT,*
GCS (Geriatric Certified Specialist), MEd

WHEELING & DEALING

WHEELING & DEALING

A Guidebook for Travelers with Disabilities

[signatures]

Sue Maris Allen, MPH, MSW

The Reverend
Barbara Ramnaraine, B.A.

SEABOARD PRESS
JAMES A. ROCK & COMPANY, PUBLISHERS

Wheeling & Dealing: A Guidebook for Travelers with Disabilities
by Sue Maris Allen and Barbara Ramnaraine

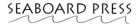

is an imprint of JAMES A. ROCK & CO., PUBLISHERS

Wheeling & Dealing: A Guidebook for Travelers with Disabilities
copyright ©2008 by Sue Maris Allen and Barbara Ramnaraine

Special contents of this edition copyright ©2008 by Seaboard Press

All applicable copyrights and other rights reserved worldwide. No part of
this publication may be reproduced, in any form or by any means,
for any purpose, except as provided by the U.S. Copyright Law,
without the express, written permission of the publisher.

Note: Product names, logos, brands, and other trademarks occurring or referred
to within this work are the property of their respective trademark holders.

Cover Design by Kippie Palesch, Minneapolis, MN
kpalesch@gmail.com

Address comments and inquiries to:
SEABOARD PRESS
9710 Traville Gateway Drive, #305
Rockville, MD 20850

E-mail:
jrock@rockpublishing.com   lrock@rockpublishing.com
Internet URL: www.rockpublishing.com

Trade Paperback ISBN: 978-1-59663-796-2

Library of Congress Control Number: 2007928325

Printed in the United States of America

First Edition: 2008

*This book is dedicated to my children and my mentors.
They have put up with my foibles, celebrated my
successes, and enriched my life immensely.
—Barbara Ramnaraine*

*To my great-grandmother, Nancy Jane Kepp Bryant, who at age
ninety filled my toddler years with stories, songs and games. A
stroke survivor and wheelchair user, she
traveled with me as far as our imaginations reached.
Only as an adult did I realize that this woman,
who taught me life's joys, was a
person with a disability.
—Sue Maris Allen*

*And, to the fifty million-plus persons with disabilities,
who travel or are considering the possibility
of traveling, we dedicate this book.
—Barbara and Sue*

ACKNOWLEDGMENTS

We are grateful to our many friends, professional colleagues and relatives who have expressed interest and encouragement in making this project come true. All have shared their unique talents generously and willingly.

Especially we thank those who reviewed our manuscript at its various stages and provided suggestions:

Richard Allen for his legal advice and tireless efforts in reading each version of the manuscript and his continuing support to both of us.

James R Allen, MD, neurological consultant and former President, Minneapolis Clinic of Neurology (ret); M.A. Blake; Robin Titterington, recipient of two prestigious awards presented by ALDA (Association for Late Deafened Adults) and Professor Nancy Eustis, both of whom provided tips for wheelchair users; Shelly Watkins; Catherine Senne Wallace; Mary Maris Watkins, and also to Lisa TenBarge PT, DPT and Kathleen Ganley, PhD for their advice and professional knowledge of Physical Therapy.

To those whose anecdotes enriched the text: Jim Hallenberg; Virginia Ott, septuagenarian and author; Jeffrey Shaw; Stephen Venable; and Janice Parker.

To those who offered professional advice and resources: Billie Howard, renowned photographer specializing in health, and his wife Laurie Shock, exhibitors of photographs of those who are blind or visually impaired; Kent Collins, Doctor of Audiology; Julie Aman Allen for her library research and her husband, Jerry Aman, for his special knowledge of adapted vehicles; and Jean Forrey.

To Carol Nulsen, friend and writing colleague, who has unselfishly shared her time and ideas and introduced us to community leaders who are advocates for persons with disabilities.

To Marc Nieson, whose patience and sensitivity to our book's mission provided encouragement that the right publisher would bring it into a book format.

To Estalita Slivoskey, who guided us through the indexing process.

To the Rock Publishers: Jim and Lynne Rock and Lilda RockWiley who, from the beginning, provided support and enthusiasm for our book.

And, our deep gratitude goes especially to our families whose support has made it a family affair. To Amy Ramnaraine who offered practical and sage advice for the book's proposed format; James Ramnaraine, who shared anecdotes and Margaret Ramnaraine who shared her knowledge of technology. To Melissa Allen, who read the manuscript and guided us with her legal expertise in copyright law; Christopher Allen, who spent hours designing our web site; and Maris Allen Venable, who reviewed the manuscript, helped us network and shared her expertise in marketing.

CONTENTS

Introduction xv

CHAPTER 1
FLYING BLIND 1
   Barbara's Tale 1
   Sue's Tale 3
   Minimizing Flight Fright 5
      The Squeaky Wheel 5
      It's in the Timing 6
      Head of the Line 6
   A Note about Preboarding 7

CHAPTER 2
RULES AS TOOLS, The Air Carrier Access Act 9
   A Helping Hand 9
   Seating Denied? Get It in Writing 10
   Qualifying For The FAA EXIT ROWS 11
   Leaving Passengers Unattended 13
   Giving Advance Notice 13
   Travel with Groups of Ten or More 14
   Traveling with A Personal Care Attendant (PCA) 15
   Travel with Service Animals 16
   This Is Your Captain Speaking 16
   Making Your Complaints Known 17
   Future Changes 18

CHAPTER 3
THE UPS AND DOWNS
OF FLYING, Becoming the Savvy Airline Traveler 21
   Plane Talk 21
   Book Early 21

Choose Electronic Tickets (e-tickets) 22
Confirm Your Reservation 23
Print-out Your Boarding Pass 23
Decode The Airport/City Codes 23
Selecting Your Flights:
   Non-Stop, Direct, or Connect 24
Direct Flights 24
Connecting Flights 25
Check-In: Curbside or Ticket Counter 27
Beverages and Snacks 28
Requesting a Wheelchair at the Terminal 28
Security 101 29
   Surgically Implanted Devices 30
   Pacemaker/Defibrillator 30
   Cochlear Implants 30
Point of No Return 31
Shoes 32
Service Animals and Security 32
Hard-of-Hearing Passengers 33
Safety Briefings 33
Keep It Light 34
Medical Oxygen 34
Food on Board 35
Arrival Procedures 37
Motorized Wheelchairs or Scooters 38
   Wheelchair Batteries 39
   Spillable Wet Cell Batteries 39
   Non-Spillable Dry Cell, Gel-Cell Batteries 40
   Do Not Drain the Battery 40
   Packaging a Disconnected Battery 40

Other Assistive Devises 40
Current and Future Findings 41
    Prohibited Items 41
    Checkpoint 41
    Kiosks 42
Food and Beverages 42
Frequent Flyer Miles 42
Changing Rules 43

CHAPTER 4
ALL ABOARD: Get on Track with Amtrak 45
    Accessible Amtrak Stations 46
    Purchase Tickets 47
    Charge To Your Credit Card 48
    Accessible Passenger Cars 49
        Accessible Bedrooms 50
        Available Equipment 50
        Accessible Space 51
        Reserve Accessible Space 51
        "Hold" Accessible Bedroom 52
        Accessible Seating in Club Cars 52
    Carry-On And Checked Baggage 52
    Railway Discount Fares 53
    No Double Dipping 53
    No Smoking 54
    Travel with Your Service Animal 54
    Food Service 54
    Medical Oxygen 56

CHAPTER 5
TRAVELING BY MOTOR COACH 59
    Speaking of Greyhound 59

No Reservations Policy 60
Ticketing 60
    "Will Call" 60
    Tickets by Mail 61
    Tickets at the Greyhound Agency 61
    Tickets by phone 61
    Discounted fares 61
Greyhound Disabilities Assist Line 62
Accessible Equipment 62
Guidelines for Traveling on Greyhound 63
    Arrive and Check-in Early 63
    Assist Passengers Boarding 63
    Assistive Devices 63
    Checked and Carry-On 64
    Baggage 64
    Questions and Prohibited Items 65
    Medical Information 65
    Medical Oxygen 65
    No Smoking 66
    Personal Identification 66
    Priority Seating 66
    Proof-of-Disability 66
    Personal Care Attendant (PCA) 66
    Sample Guidelines for PCA Program 67
    Trained Service Animals 68
    Travel with a Minor 68
Food Service and Greyhound 69
Submit Your Complaints 69

CHAPTER 6
GET SMARTER WHEN YOU CHARTER 71
    The Bus, Van or Other Vehicle 72

The Company 73
The Driver 73
Insurance 74
Insurance Coverage 74
References 74
Safety Rating 74
Special Needs for Travelers with Disabilities 74
Subcontracting Agreements 75

CHAPTER 7
TAKE A BRAKE 77

CHAPTER 8
PUTTING IT ALL TOGETHER! 81
Juggling Your Way Through the Terminal 81
Packing Light 82
    Baggage 83
    Shoes 84
    Heavy coat or jacket 85
    Books or recorded books 85
Medicines and Medical Equipment 86
    Documenting your health 86
        1. Personal identification documents 87
        2. Electronic devices 87
        3. Medical documents 88
        4. Insurance documents 89
Carry-on and Checked Baggage 92
    Carry-on bags 92
    Tips for diabetics 93
Guard your Security 93
Travel and Food 94
    Airlines 95

    Amtrak 95
    Automobile 95
    Greyhound 96
  A Little Extra Assist 96
    Airlines 97
    Travel with your powered wheelchair 97
  Handling Wheelchair Batteries 98
    Spillable wet cell batteries 98
    Non-spillable dry cell, gel-cell batteries 98
    Do not drain the battery 99
    Packaging a disconnected battery 99

CHAPTER 9
LET THE JOURNEY BEGIN 101

Endnotes 103
References and Resources 105
Major Domestic (US) Airlines 109
Major Domestic Airport Codes 111
Checklist for Packing 113
Checklist for Packing for Trip 114
My List of Items to Pack 115
About the Authors
  Sue Maris Allen. MSW 117
  The Reverand Barbara Ramnaraine. BA 119
Index 121

INTRODUCTION

Disabilities can happen at anytime. A permanent disability or a temporary limitation can result from a health condition, an automobile accident, a plummet down a ski slope or a slip in the bathtub. Any of us, at some time in our life, may find ourselves dealing with a disability. Yet such situations shouldn't necessarily hamper our mobility or our dreams to travel. Persons with disabilities should expect to receive the kind of carefree travel that able-bodied travelers experience.

We speak with the authority that comes from experiencing, living and traveling years with our own disabilities. We have traveled thousands of miles alone and with our families. Most of our travels have been happy, but a few left us feeling frustrated. In the following pages, we share our travel experiences, the good times and the disappointments.

Although our perspectives frequently come from visual disabilities, Sue also experiences the challenges of coronary artery disease, diabetes, osteoporosis and rehabilitation following strokes. In addition to Retinitis Pigmentosa, Barbara also experienced a hip replacement. Our suggestions, therefore, aim to reflect and support the needs of travelers with diverse disabilities. This book is for you and the fifty million-plus persons with disabilities who travel, or are considering the possibility of travel. It is to all of you that we offer the information in this book and hope you too will find it useful.

We begin by relating incidents that have occurred to us as we traveled separately across the country at different times and for different purposes. Throughout the book you will find anecdotes preceded by our initials (BR for Barbara; SMA for Sue) and accented with italicized type. Some come from our own experiences, others have been shared by friends and family members. Initially you may find these tales discouraging. Read on. Our stories do have a happy ending. We enjoy traveling and we thank all the employees of the airlines, the buses, chartered buses and trains who provide all of us with the support and care we need.

CHAPTER 1

FLYING BLIND

Barbara's Tale

I have *Retinitis Pigmentosa*, a condition that clouds the retina and prevents images from reaching the vision center of the brain. For the first 27 years of my life I was "legally blind" yet able to move around without a white cane and able to read magnified print. For over 40 years I have had no vision at all. During this period I raised my children and made a career shift to become a deacon in the Episcopal Church. For about 15 years, I have traveled regularly throughout the country as a member of a taskforce for my church. I have always used the same air carrier because they have served me well and provided the assistance I needed. Most of the time I travel alone and have a friend or business colleague meet me at my destination.

In July 2000, I attended our church's convention in Denver. My usual practice when flying is to alert the reservationist when I schedule my flight, mentioning that I need assistance in boarding and deplaning. I followed this practice when I made my July flight.

After arriving in Denver, one of the flight attendants was walking with me from the plane to the gate where I was going to be met by a long time friend, when an airport employee pushing two wheelchairs stopped us.

"I've been instructed to take you in a wheelchair," he said.

I tried to explain to him that someone was meeting me and that we had only a few feet left to walk.

"No," he insisted rather aggressively, "You must ride in the wheelchair."

And so, I complied. When we had gone further than I thought the gate should be, I reminded him I was meeting someone at the gate.

"There's no one at the gate," he said.

He continued rolling me through the terminal, finally arriving at what I sensed from the echoes was a large, concrete corridor with few people. He stopped, and told me that he was taking the other woman, whose chair he was also pushing, to her gate.

"But my friend can't find me in this area," I said. "Please, I want to go to the airline's check-in desk."

"You are selfish and only thinking of yourself. Like in the military, when a command is given, it must be obeyed unless it is countermanded by the person who issued the order."

He left me sitting in the middle of nowhere, alone and disoriented, and not knowing how to get to the airline reservation desk or how to get back to the gate.

I waited fifteen to twenty minutes. No one approached me. No one came within shouting distance. Nor did I perceive anyone within the vicinity. Then, I began to hear my name being called to go to a courtesy phone for a message. I had no idea where the courtesy phone was, so I continued to sit. Finally, after another ten minutes or so, an airport employee approached.

"Do you need any help?"

"Yes, I have a friend meeting me but I can't get to the courtesy phone to let her know where I am."

He took me to a courtesy phone and within minutes my friend found me. She was frantic; I was livid.

Though I was not hurt physically, my confidence in my ability to fly independently was sorely compromised. I was angry because I wasn't listened to and because I was forced to use a wheelchair when I was perfectly able to walk with minimal assistance.

After several phone calls and a letter to the president of the airlines, I received a compensatory travel voucher and a letter of apology. These incidents should not have happened, but too often similar incidents do occur. As you will see, they are in clear violation of the Air Carrier Access Act. This book is our attempt to help you avoid some of the anxiety that such a situation can evoke.

Sue's Tale

I had given little thought to traveling as a passenger with a disability. I assumed that I always would be able-bodied. In 1999, however, I experienced visual and other impairments caused by strokes.

Soon thereafter my sisters invited me to visit them for a special celebration in Arizona and I questioned my ability to make the trip alone. Would someone assist me through a bustling airport or guide me from the boarding gate to the door of the plane? Would I find my assigned seat on the plane? My anxiety mounted in those days before the flight.

At that time, my friend Barbara, a clergy person on the staff at our church, had been blind for many years. She'd spoken to me with self-assurance about her previous travel experiences.

Based on her advice, I made my airline reservation well in advance of the scheduled flight, and informed the reservations agent about my limited vision. The agent, too, was reassuring. She told me she was entering a request for assistance in her computer's data bank. This meant that other employees, seeing the entry, would realize they should help me board and deplane.

When my travel date finally arrived, my trepidations were confirmed. At my boarding gate, the gate attendant appeared skeptical when I reminded him that I needed assistance walking down the jetway to the plane. He frowned and told me to step aside while he helped other passengers. When all other passengers had boarded, he seemed to follow me reluctantly down the ramp toward the outbound flight.

Unfairly, I questioned my own behavior. Was I doing something wrong? Surely these employees helped passengers with disabilities every day. Why was I put in a position of feeling failure and rejection for merely asking for assistance? Where were those friendly skies Barbara had described?

Those friendly skies arrived 1200 miles away in the person of a wheelchair attendant. She immediately conveyed an attitude of confident support. She suggested that the distance from the gate to the parking ramp required use of a wheelchair (and she was right). She willingly pushed the heavy wheelchair through an "under construction" airport, and insisted that she wait with me until my sister and her friend arrived.

I anticipated the same supportive experience on my return flight from Phoenix a week later. It was not to be. My niece asked the gate attendant for help when I was ready to board the plane. The attendant avoided speaking directly to me, and addressed my niece in a dismissive voice, "It isn't far. They won't let her sit in the wrong seat." Fortunately, a concerned passenger followed me down the aisle and helped me locate my seat. His kindness placed me in the right row, but on the wrong side of the aisle! This time I didn't feel vulnerable, but duly frustrated and ignored.

Minimizing Flight Fright

Since these incidents occurred, we've learned to be more proactive and more savvy, while remaining flexible and open to changes, in order to enjoy a safe and pleasant trip. We have paid special attention to adjusting our preboarding and deplaning habits. Here are a few tips we both observe:

The Squeaky Wheel

Most of us have heard that "the squeaky wheel gets the oil." Airline employees deal with many passengers and hear many "squeaky wheels" in a given day. We need to remind them of our specific needs so they can respond as quickly as possible. When asked to step aside until others have been helped, as happened to Sue, we describe our special need to the gate attendant and our request for preboarding. By telling the attendant or other employee about our needs, we provide them with information that helps them respond with the appropriate assistance.

In other words, serve as your own advocate. Just because your disability doesn't require use of a wheelchair or service animal, doesn't mean your disability should become invisible and go unnoticed. Take pride in the degree of independence you have achieved, but be realistic about the help you need.

It's in the Timing

All commercial airlines ask you to allow extra time in arriving at the terminal. Lines have grown longer for curbside check-in as well as at the ticket counter and security checkpoints. Contact your airline to find out the amount of time you should allow for arriving at the terminal for your specific flight. If the airline suggests arriving two hours prior to departure, clarify whether you should be at curbside check-in, waiting in line for the security inspection, or at the boarding gate two hours before your plane's departure. Parking, traffic or unanticipated incidents can cause delays. Factor these unexpected events into your timetable. You will feel less stressed and less hurried when you allow extra time for making your way through the terminal and reaching your boarding gate. In turn, unhurried airline employees will be able to give you and any equipment you're carrying its deserved attention.

Head of the Line

When you arrive at the boarding gate, sit near the door where passengers for your flight board. If you are unsure which door leads to your flight, ask one of the attendants at the desk. When the boarding gate attendant announces boarding time for those passengers traveling with children or needing extra time in boarding, you can easily step to the head of the line. Explain to the gate attendants that you are concerned about being inadvertently bumped or pushed out of the way by passengers rushing to find seats or stow items in the overhead bins. Passengers with disabilities often find it easier to be first in line to preboard.

A Note about Preboarding

Although many airlines offer preboarding privileges, the FAA does not require them to do so. Among those airlines (such as some discounted airlines) that do not offer preboarding on a regular basis, passengers with disabilities should be granted that privilege, if they arrive at the boarding gate early and request preboarding. Call your airline and ask about their preboarding policy.

Becoming a savvy and safe traveler requires planning, flexibility and confidence in your own abilities. Current events mandate frequent changes in rules and regulations pertaining to security and public transportation. We recommend that you contact the Department of Transportation (DOT) www.dot.gov, Federal Aviation Administration (FAA) www.faa.gov, Transportation Security Administration (TSA) www.tsa.gov or your carrier for updated information.

Our purpose for writing this book is two-fold. First, we want to provide you with the tools to minimize travel terrors. Second, whether you have a new disability or whether you have lived with your disability all your life, or whether you're traveling on business or for pleasure, we want to help enhance and preserve your confidence. We hope that the following pages will provide you with a fair measure of each.

CHAPTER 2

RULES AS TOOLS
The Air Carrier Access Act

All airlines are responsible for the safety and comfort of their passengers. This responsibility includes passengers with disabilities just as it does able-bodied passengers. Further, the Air Carrier Access Act (ACAA),[1] requires that air carriers cannot, by law, discriminate against passengers with disabilities. We have listed below some of the ACAA rules the airlines must follow in order to meet federal laws. We suggest you become familiar with them so you will know your rights and what you should expect from the airlines. At the same time, you also need to know the nature of *your* responsibility to the airlines. You can obtain the ACAA's complete list of rules in the Department of Transportation's booklet, "New Horizons: Information for the Air Traveler with a Disability."[2] You can download this at the DOT website (See References and Resources).

A Helping Hand

Under federal rules, the air carrier is required to offer help to a passenger with a disability when they are boarding or deplaning. (See ACAA RULE)

Many passengers with disabilities are unaware that responsibility to provide assistance in boarding and deplaning rests with the airlines.

Personal Experiences

SMA: My daughter, scheduled on a flight connecting in North Carolina, was required to make an unexpected transfer to a second plane. All the passengers walked several feet outdoors in a light rain from one plane and climbed a metal stairway to board the connecting flight. My daughter followed a passenger who was carrying a young child with a disability. The young mother struggled with her child and a collapsible child's stroller, as she made her way up the metal stairs. The airline employees did not offer assistance to any of the passengers.

BR: Traveling with a different airline, I once found myself in a similar situation, yet airline attendants were waiting at the metal stairway ready to provide assistance to anyone in need.

Seating Denied? Get It in Writing

Airlines cannot refuse you a seat on a flight only because of your disability. If you are excluded from the flight based on your disability, they must explain the reason, and send you a written explanation within ten (10) calendar days. (See: ACAA RULE)

The airline cannot deny you a seat on your flight based *only* on your disability. However, they can refuse you transportation if your disability would either: 1) endanger the health or safety of other passengers, or, 2) would violate FAA safety rules. The airline must, however, provide transportation to persons whose disabilities may affect their involuntary behavior or their personal appearance (e.g., Parkinson's or Turret's Syndrome).[3] In some situations the airline can deny you transportation for a reason separate from your disability. You may have told crew members (or they might suspect) that you are ill with a communicable disease. Diseases such as SARS or Small Pox, for example, can spread from passenger to passenger and can cause the airline to act out of concern for your health and safety and the health and safety of *all* their passengers by denying you transportation. If your physician has given you a statement indicating that your condition is not presently communicable, or has been treated and cannot be passed from you to other passengers, submit that medical statement to your airline. A carrier excluding you from a flight for safety reasons *must* tell you the reason(s). And, they must follow-up with a written explanation of their action within ten calendar days.

Qualifying For The FAA EXIT ROWS

Airlines must assign you the seat of your choice (with the exception of the FAA EXIT ROW), unless the seat you request has been previously assigned to another passenger. (See ACAA RULE)

The Federal Aviation Administration (FAA) sets aside certain rows on each flight to be designated as FAA EXIT ROWS. They are marked with the word EXIT in red above that row of seats. For your safety, ask an attendant to point out the EXIT rows. Passengers sitting in these seats must be able to provide help to other passengers in case of an emergency landing. The passenger sitting next to the window in this EXIT row must be able to:

1. Read the instructions for opening the aircraft's emergency door, (both see the instructions as well as read the language);
2. Open the *heavy* EMERGENCY DOOR EXIT door;
3. Assist passengers exiting the plane; and
4. Remain calm and composed during an emergency.

You may never be called on to perform these tasks, but accepting a seat in a designated FAA EXIT row does carry these potential responsibilities. If your disability prevents you from performing these obligations, inform the airline and don't allow them to assign you an FAA EXIT row seat.

In the world today, the threat of terrorism requires that all passengers remain flexible. Carriers can initiate changes quickly demanding that all of us respond to new seating patterns, limit carry-on baggage, or restrict other items carried on board the flight.

Except for the designated FAA EXIT row, the airlines must make an effort to give you the seat of your choice. Of course, if the seat has been previously assigned to another passenger, the attendant is not required to ask that passenger to move. Airlines may require that you request your preferred seat 48-hours before departure, and that you check-in 90-minutes prior to boarding. Call your carrier a few days before your scheduled flight to confirm their rules about check-in time and when you must request your preferred seat.

Leaving Passengers Unattended

A carrier cannot leave a passenger, who is not independently mobile, unattended for more than 30 minutes. (See ACAA RULE)

If you use a wheelchair, crutches or other assistive device, your carrier cannot leave you unattended for a period of more than 30-minutes, unless you are independently mobile.

Personal Experiences

BR: You will recall from Chapter 1 that I am blind and was left unattended in a ground wheelchair in the Denver airport. If you file a formal complaint, as I did, be aware that complaints also should be filed with the wheelchair vendors directly. Airports or airlines often contract with independent vendors who employ the wheelchair attendants.

Giving Advance Notice

Except in specific situations, the airlines cannot require you, a person with a disability, to inform them that you will be traveling with them or of your disability. (See: ACAA RULE)

Many passengers with disabilities are able to check-in and board without additional help from airline employees. However, most find it prudent to inform the airline about the nature of their disability. Telling the reservation agent, the gate attendant, and the cabin attendant "I have low vision," or "I'm a wheelchair user," or carrying a written note stating "I'm hard-of-hearing" gives the airline employees an opportunity to give you extra attention. If you make your reservation online, some airlines provide a question for you to answer indicating your special needs. Although we recommend that persons with disabilities disclose any special need for safety reasons, the airline cannot require you to do so.

Personal Experiences

SMA: An airline representative in Arizona told my niece that I should have given the airline advance notice that I have a visual impairment. In fact, I told the reservation agent when I purchased my ticket that I would need assistance boarding and deplaning. However, the airline cannot require advance notice.

There are times, such as in the following situations, you will *need* to give advance notice.

1. If the carrier needs time to prepare for a passenger's accommodation (supplying oxygen for you, for example), or
2. If the aircraft has fewer than 60 seats and is carrying your powered wheelchair, the airline may require you to give up to 48-hours notice.
3. Whenever you are unsure about informing your carrier in advance about your special needs, it is best to do so.

Travel with Groups of Ten or More

The airline cannot limit the number of persons with disabilities traveling in your group. However, if your group exceeds ten (10), some rules apply, see paragraph below. (See: ACAA RULE)

Groups, such as churches, schools, scouts and other organizations often want to travel together for enjoyment, efficiency and economy. Air carriers cannot impose a limit on the number of persons with disabilities traveling on a flight. The airline may require, however, that you notify them up to 48-hours in advance of your trip, if ten or more of you travel in a group. You also can assist both your group and your airline if you ask your airline to help you estimate the amount of time you will need for boarding. Tell them your flight number and the number of persons with disabilities traveling with you. Request your gate number and confirm it at the terminal.

Traveling with A Personal Care Attendant (PCA)

A carrier may require a Personal Care Attendant (PCA) to travel with persons who may not understand instructions or are unable to assist in their evacuation from the aircraft because of their disability. If the passenger and aircraft personnel disagree about the need for a PCA, the air carrier can require a PCA, but cannot charge the passenger or the Personal Care Attendant for the attendant's transportation. (See: ACAA RULE)

Your air carrier cannot require you to travel with a Personal Care Attendant (PCA) *solely* because you are a passenger with a disability. Airline personnel may express concern for your overall safety if you or other passengers might have difficulty following instructions in safely evacuating the plane in the event of an emergency. The airline can challenge your decision to travel without a Personal Care Attendant. If you and your airline cannot reach an agreement about your need for a Personal Care Attendant (PCA), the airline can require you to travel with a PCA. The airline, however, cannot charge you or your Personal Care Attendant for the attendant's fare when the airline makes the decision. If you have any doubt about your need for a Personal Care Attendant, ask your physician's advice when planning your trip.

Travel with Service Animals

Carriers must allow service animals to accompany a person with a disability on a flight, provided the service animal has credible documentation, a harness, tags or other appropriate identification. (See: ACAA RULE)

Airlines must permit your *trained* Service animal to accompany you and cannot deny you any seat (except the FAA EXIT ROW or a previously assigned seat) unless your Service animal obstructs an aisle or other area that must remain clear in case of an emergency. Service animals must have appropriate identification, which can include documentation and a harness. *Note:* At the time of this writing, these ACAA Rules are being studied and this is one of the rules that may be revised. Several changes are under consideration, but to our knowledge a decision has not been made. Check the www.faa.gov website for changes.

This Is Your Captain Speaking

Carriers must provide travel information (on such items as ticketing, changes in schedule) to passengers with disabilities in a manner as timely as provided to able-bodied passengers. (See: ACAA RULE)

All information relating to flight status changes must be available to passengers, regardless of any disabilities, and should be provided in a format passengers can use. For example, passengers who are deaf or cannot speak may need to communicate through written notes. If you cannot understand announcements from the pilot, the gate attendant or cabin attendant, or other personnel, *ask*. You should receive these details at your request. This includes information alerting you to changes such as gate assignments, luggage check-in, schedule changes, status of your flight ticketing (has there been a change?) and weather alerts (e.g., turbulence).

Making Your Complaints Known

At least one Complaints Resolution Official (CRO) must be available for each carrier at each airport during scheduled operations. Passengers having complaints of violation of the ACAA rules have the right to communicate with the CRO. (See: ACAA RULE)

Disputes occasionally occur between a passenger with a disability and the airline. Each airline must provide at least one Complaints Resolution Officer (CRO) at each airport to help settle disagreements relating to your disability. The CRO must be available at the airport during scheduled hours of operation, and must be on the premises, or, if necessary, may be contacted by phone. The CRO is given the authority to decide disputes on behalf of the carrier. Passengers who are not satisfied with the decision can contact the Department of Transportation. The DOT urges you to report violations of the ACAA at the hotline 1-800-778-4838 (phone) or 1-800-455-9880 (TTY). Phone lines are staffed from 7:00

a.m. to 11:00 p.m. ET (at this writing). If you want the complaint investigated further, put it in writing, and address it to the Department of Transportation. Pertinent addresses, Websites for downloading a Complaint form, or Toll-Free numbers for requesting a Complaint form can be found in the References and Resources section.

Personal Experiences

BR: The Department of Transportation (DOT) regularly investigates the number of complaints filed against each airline. Although I did not contact DOT when my airline left me stranded, they nevertheless learned of this incident on their own. Consequently, I was contacted by DOT and asked if I would be a part of an action which they were bringing against that airline. Too many complaints had been lodged by persons with disabilities, and DOT wanted to correct this situation. When finally the case was settled, the airline was assessed a considerable penalty and directed to correct the situations for which the case had been initiated.

Each of us, I believe, owes it to ourselves and all other people with disabilities who now fly or who may fly in the future to make the airlines know when our rights have been violated.

Future Changes

The Department of Transportation once again is studying these rules and two rules outlined in this chapter are subject to change. As we mentioned earlier in this chapter, one rule relates to transporting service animals. The second change would require airlines to provide respiratory services for passengers who require medical oxygen. At this writing, these changes have not become law. Contact the Department of Transportation (www.dot.gov) or refer to ACAA changes online.

CHAPTER 3

THE UPS AND DOWNS OF FLYING
Becoming the Savvy Airline Traveler

Plane Talk

Following the tragic events of September 11, 2001, we've all become more alert and more cautious travelers. Our willingness to put safety ahead of our personal comfort is demonstrated daily as we wait in line for security guards to check our personal identification, scan us with metal detector wands and inspect our baggage. Tips that always have been good practices for passengers with disabilities now have become essential for the sake of safety, efficiency and comfort. We have selected, in the following paragraphs, a few tips that may help even out the ups and downs of our flight experiences, and provide smoother trips.

Book Early

You don't want to miss important board meetings, scheduled business conferences, Aunt Hannah's eightieth birthday celebration, or religious holidays with your family. And, you want to get the best possible fare. Whether for business or pleasure, reserve space on your flight early. Passengers with disabilities recognize the importance of reserving travel space weeks, or sometimes months before their scheduled departure. One airline advises to plan months ahead if you need to travel on a specific, unchangeable date. Early booking may seem unnecessary, but remember that the best fares and seat assignments will be based on availability.

Choose Electronic Tickets (e-tickets)

Without leaving home, you can charge your airline ticket, confirm your reservation, print out your boarding pass and select your preferred seat, all through the Internet on your personal computer. Additionally, the Internet offers you the opportunity to browse for the best fare, create your personal itinerary, describe your special needs (e.g., low vision or hard-of-hearing) and request your personal options, such as seat selection. Although paper tickets can be purchased through your airline ticket office, your travel agent or requested by phone or online, most airlines now charge an extra fee for paper tickets. Some airlines predict that paper tickets will be unavailable within a short time.

Your e-ticket will eliminate the need for a paper ticket, and free you from spending anxious days waiting for its arrival by U.S. mail. And, you can avoid searching for it just before you head to the airport. You can thus avoid longer lines at the check-in counter and move more quickly through security checkpoints. A separate ticket line is designated at most airports for passengers holding e-tickets, or you can use the freestanding automatic kiosk positioned in many terminals. Pick-up your boarding pass at the kiosk if you haven't already done so through your personal computer. You may need to use your credit card (for identification) to swipe through the slot provided for that purpose at the ticket counter or kiosk.

Confirm Your Reservation

Your confirmation number will be issued to you when you make your reservation, and is a combination of letters and numbers (#12AQ45, for example). Hold onto it. Whether you book by phone or Internet, put a copy of that number in a safe place. And *remember where you put it*. The airlines will match you to your ticket through this confirmation number each time you contact them about any detail of your flight. Make certain a written summary of your airline reservations and itinerary are sent to you by e-mail or U.S. mail. Look over the itinerary and the reservations as soon as you receive them. Contact your airline or travel agent immediately about any mistake in the flight numbers, dates, times or cities of departure or arrival. Yes, you will need to provide your confirmation number.

Print-out Your Boarding Pass

Most airlines encourage you to print-out your Boarding Pass from your personal computer prior to leaving home. You can print it out as early as 24-hours before your scheduled flight. Unless you need to check baggage, you can go directly to the security line and the boarding gate, presenting your Boarding Pass to the agents at those check points.

Decode The Airport/City Codes

You won't need a decoder ring to identify airport codes throughout the country. Use the list of cities in the United

States with major airports listed in the Major Domestic Airport Codes section to identify each airport by its three-letter code. Minneapolis-St. Paul, for example, is listed as MSP, and Phoenix as PHX. Larger cities, such as Chicago, can be the home of more than one major airport. You will find these listings quicker and more convenient if you use their 3-letter code. For example, Chicago-O'Hare uses ORD and Chicago-Midway uses MDW; Los Angeles uses LAX, but Burbank, also in the Los Angeles area, is noted as BUR. Watch for those 3-letters on luggage tags and tickets. Although knowing your Airport Code isn't mandatory at the present time, using it will prove faster and more efficient when confirming or reserving your ticket online, or filling out a baggage form.

Selecting Your Flights: Non-Stop, Direct, or Connect

Travelers with disabilities will feel less stressed by scheduling on Non-Stop flights, when possible. Non-stop flights, take-off from City A (Minneapolis, for example) and land at City B (Nashville, for example). There are no stops between City A (Minneapolis) and City B (Nashville). Checked or carry-on baggage and equipment such as a powered wheelchair, stay on the plane with you until you reach your final destination.

Direct Flights

The term "direct flight" refers to a modification of the Non-Stop flight. Suppose you fly from City A (Minneapolis) to City B (Detroit) non-stop, where other passengers will board and deplane. After landing at City B, you will stay on the same plane and fly on to your final destination, City C

(Nashville). Passengers continuing on to City C (Nashville, for example) *will not* change aircraft before reaching their final destination. Checked or carry-on baggage or special equipment will remain on the plane with you during your stop over in City B (Detroit).

> *Personal Experiences*
>
> *BR & SMA: As passengers with disabilities, both of us find it less tiring and less stressful to book our flights on a non-stop or direct flight. We urge you to consider following this same practice, even though the fare may be more expensive. Discount agencies frequently offer lower ticket fares for either direct or connecting flights. I have purchased tickets from such agencies as Hotwire, Orbitz or Priceline and have always received a bargain price, but my connecting airport can be as close to my home airport (Minneapolis-St. Paul) as Chicago or as out-of-the-way as Cincinnati or Dallas.*

Connecting Flights

If you book connecting flights, expect to make one or more stops and *change planes* at least once between your departure and final destination. Passengers, their baggage and their equipment (powered wheel chairs or other assistive devices), *will change* aircraft at each stop. Boarding gates for connecting flights can be located a few steps away or sometimes they can be more than a mile apart. When using a connecting flight, allow adequate time for deplaning and finding the gate for your next outbound flight. We mention allowing adequate time because of the many variables involved. Usually allow a minimum of 1-1/2 to 2-hours. The numbers of passengers in security lines and the distance from the entrance of the terminal to the boarding gate must be taken into account.

Passengers boarding at Los Angeles LAX, for example, may need more time than those boarding at Des Moines, Iowa. Those of us with disabilities must allow for our particular needs. If you have assistive devices with you, inform the agent helping confirm your reservation. Your wheelchair, baggage and other checked equipment stowed in the cargo bin of your connecting flight should be transferred for you. You will be responsible for transferring any carry-on items.

Personal Experiences

SMA: My husband and I were booked on a flight connecting in Chicago O'Hare (ORD). My impaired vision and my husband's recent heart attack required that we each reserve a wheelchair. The reservation agent assured us that the wheelchairs would be waiting for us when we arrived in Chicago. He also told us that one hour between flights would provide adequate time to make our connection. We arrived in Chicago to find 1) no wheelchairs and 2) a trek of 1-1/4 miles between gates. We phoned for the wheelchairs and they arrived with only thirty minutes to roll us through the airport. The attendant who pushed my wheelchair seemed exhausted as she pushed my 135-pounds. (I was more stressed about her physical condition than about missing my plane.) She finally met another wheelchair attendant (this one probably played football in his off-duty time) and she breathlessly asked him to roll my wheelchair the rest of the dis-

tance. He obliged and we arrived at the gate of our outbound flight with only minutes to spare.

Yes, we saved money on the connecting flight, but we paid the difference in stress and worry. Even though many of us feel able to walk the mile or so from one gate to another under ordinary circumstances, we may want to accept the ride in a wheelchair or shuttle car as a concession to our own independence.

Check-In: Curbside or Ticket Counter

Your attention to security begins before you leave home. Think through what you are taking onboard. Lists of items you cannot bring to a security check point and into the airline cabin are available through the Transportation Security Administration (TSA) and can be found online at www.tsa.gov. Changes can occur frequently, and we urge that you check with both TSA and your carrier for allowed and prohibited items.

The Transportation Security Administration (TSA) (www.tsa.gov) on their website, presents the 3-1-1 icon to help remember the rule to carry-on liquids, gels and toiletries:

1. Pack liquid, gels and aerosols in containers of 3-ounces or less.
2. Place these containers in a 1-quart-size, clear plastic sealeable bag. Gallon-size bags, or bags that do not provide a sealeable closure are not allowed.
3. Only one plastic bag is allowed per passenger in a *carry-on* bag. You may carry-on certain excep-

tions such as prescription and non-prescription medicines, baby formula, breast milk, and baby food while traveling with a baby or small child. Liquids (such as water and juice) also may be carried for medical conditions (diabetes, for example). You must declare such items to a Security Officer during screening.

Beverages and Snacks

Coffee, sodas and other similar items may be purchased from vendors in the terminal after passing through security checkpoints. These articles can then be taken onboard your flight.

For an update on current security rules, we suggest you contact your airline or the TSA www.tsa.gov for the latest, most complete list before every flight.

Carry at least one government-issued picture Identification with you (e.g., driver's license, non-driver's license identification, passport, military I.D.) for security agents and ticket agents. You also need to carry your airline boarding pass. Only ticketed passengers can go beyond the security checkpoints.

Requesting a Wheelchair at the Terminal

If you need a wheelchair and wheelchair attendant to take you to your boarding gate, follow these steps:

1. Request a wheelchair at the time you book your flight. Your boarding pass or your ticket should indicate you have ordered a wheelchair.

2. Remind the attendant at check-in (curbside or ticket counter) that a wheelchair is assigned in your name.
3. They will page the attendant, who will bring the wheelchair to you.
4. Tell the wheelchair attendant your destination within the terminal (Gate 25, the Gold Concourse, for example) and present your ticket.
5. The wheelchair attendant will roll you first to the security check-in. Make certain your carry-on items are placed on the conveyor belt (see Security Guards and Metal Detectors, below) and moved through the metal detector.
6. The attendant will then make certain you are safely through the metal detector before undergoing inspection himself/herself.

Security 101

Upon reaching the security guards, you (both wheelchair users and mobile passengers) will be asked to empty all pockets, placing the contents in a small tray. You also will be asked to remove your belt, coat, jacket, scarves, shoes, and any other outer garments. Place these garments *and* your carry-on items in a container (a plastic bin) on a conveyer belt.

These items slowly move through a small, enclosed area for further x-ray inspection. Place coins, belts, keys and other metal objects in a small plastic container (security guards will provide these).

As your purse and your other items move along the belt, you will be asked to step through the metal detector where items such as attached metal buttons, zippers, coins, and keys can be detected by a buzzer. Metal screws and plates surgically implanted in your body also can set-off the detector's buzzer.

Surgically Implanted Devices

Metal implanted Pins, prosthetic devices, and other medical devices may cause problems at the security check. The security guard may ask to see a medical card signed by your physician, listing in detail any prosthetic devices, metal braces, metal pins, or other medical devices implanted under your skin.

Pacemaker/Defibrillator

Passengers with a pacemaker/defibrillator implant should carry an identification (ID) card, and/or consider wearing a Medic-Alert bracelet or necklace. Show the airport security officers your ID before entering the screening area since the pacemaker/defibrillator may trigger the alarm. Discuss with your physician the specific details of your implanted devise(s). Based on this information, the physician can help determine whether you should pass through the metal detector, permit the security guards to use the hand-held wand, or provide a pat-down for your security inspection.

Security guards will open your carry-on baggage and other items in order to locate the article that has tripped the metal detector. When you are asked to remove outer clothing or if you feel embarrassed with the screening, you have the right to request a private screening.

Cochlear Implants

If you have a Cochlear Implant in your ear, TSA advises it is unnecessary to remove the outer portion of the implant.

You can request an overall body search or a Pat-Down, if you do not want to go through the x-ray at the checkpoint. Some airport security guards may not be familiar with cochlear implants, so carry documentation signed by your physician, stating that you have a cochlear implant. If you use a "Hearing Dog," keep the dog with you at all times. Passengers wearing hearing aids also may alert the security guard that these devices may trip the security alarm.

Point of No Return

Once you pass through the initial inspection (x-ray and metal detector), you will enter into the "secured" area. Any person who is not ticketed is not allowed into or beyond this point of inspection. Some airports are designed so that unticketed persons will not be able to walk through or into the restaurants, food courts or other retail areas. Other terminals construct some of their restaurants and gift shops outside the secured areas, and are open to all persons visiting the terminal.

Personal Experiences

SMA: Our son-in-law phoned to tell us he would have a layover at our airport during an early morning flight. We quickly agreed to meet him during the lunch hour. Unfortunately, his flight was late, and our airport allowed no un-ticketed visitors into secured areas where all the restaurants and food courts offered meals and snacks for sale. We drove a few miles where we hurriedly ate lunch and returned to the terminal. None of us realized we would spend half our allotted time driving to and from a sandwich shop.

> *BR: My daughter and I flew to Hawaii last year. After we entered the secured area, we were told we could not leave that area for any reason. We suggest you attempt to estimate the amount of time you will be required to sit at the boarding gate once you enter that area. Ask whether food, water, and restrooms will be available in the boarding area.*

Shoes

Be prepared to remove your shoes for the security guards' inspection. Shoes with gel liners, thick soles or reinforced with metal will be carefully scrutinized since they can conceal explosives and other weapons. Shoe inspection can be one of the slowest points in the security check because putting on shoes and lacing or buckling them may require extra time. Feet can swell due to a medical condition or after a long day of walking.

Wear shoes that are large enough to slip on your feet easily after the examination. Passengers who have arthritis in their fingers or have trouble bending over may want to wear shoes that slip-on or fasten with Velcro. (see: www.tsa.gov)

Service Animals and Security

Even though airlines may accept the passenger's verbal assurance that the Service animal is trained for that purpose, a written document can avoid questions and delays. You also should carry with you the animal's health certificates and proof of vaccination. Be aware that a Service animal's collar and leash can set-off the alarm when walking through security.

Gimp-on-the-Go (www.gimponthego.com) suggests putting the Service animal (especially a service dog) at Sit-Stay with a long leash while you pass through the security gate first. You can then allow your dog to come through the gate alone, assuring the Security guards that your animal's harness is responsible for setting off the alarm. Although service dogs are commonly recognized, passengers with disabilities do bring other trained animals as well. Describe your trained animal to the airline personnel in advance of your trip. These animals will probably be allowed on the plane, but must be *trained*. Prepare to offer documentation that your animal is a *trained* service animal.

Hard-of-Hearing Passengers

Tell the airline employees, (reservation agent, ticketing agent, and the person at the boarding gate) of your specific needs.

Personal Experiences

SMA & BR: A friend of ours, who is deaf, tells us that a number of her friends avoid telling the cabin attendant that they are hard-of-hearing. Our friend, however, says she informs the attendants that she is deaf. She believes it is not only a courtesy to the attendant, but also a safety measure for her.

Safety Briefings

The airline attendants must provide a safety briefing to all passengers so they can understand the information. Safety briefing shown on a video screen must include open captions or inserts for a sign interpreter.[1] Carry with you a small note pad and pen or pencil in case you want to communicate your needs to the airline personnel, or if they want to communicate with you.

Keep It Light

A sense of humor often spans the bridge of understanding between airline employees and passengers with disabilities. Several months ago our friend's ninety-year-old relative boarded a plane in the United States bound for Canada. Her son had written a letter explaining her special needs. She presented his letter to the airline attendant. It read in part:

> *Please understand that I am deaf. I am not "hearing impaired" or any other politically correct adjective, I AM DEAF. Read the following before initiating communication: I am a U.S. Citizen. Here is my U.S. Passport and my driver's license from the State of Indiana. Yes, I know the Passport is expired. Your Customs people told my son that this would be OK as long as a valid photo ID accompanies it. I still was born on the date and in the place noted on the U.S. Passport. I am not carrying any drugs, contraband, plants, or things made out of endangered species. I have no bombs, guns, pepper-spray, or weapons of self-defense. I have no large sums of hard currency. If I did, my son would be visiting ME.*

You must share in the responsibility for meeting your needs through thoughtful planning and by developing open and honest communication with airline employees.

Medical Oxygen

Airlines are not required at the present time to offer medical oxygen on a flight. Many carriers do provide oxygen, however, if you give them 48-hour notice. (Note: The Department of Transportation is reviewing the Air Carrier Access Act and considering changing this, and other portions of the act. You are advised to watch for these decisions to be announced.) You should carry a certification of your condition from your doctor, and she/he must include a prescription for the number of liters you require per minute. Passengers cannot bring their own oxygen supply on board, and must use oxygen provided in FAA approved canisters.

> *Personal Experiences*
>
> *SMA & BR—Our friend, Jim, in his early forties, developed a temporary disability while skiing in the mountains. He phoned home to say he and his family would be delayed leaving. "I've been diagnosed with pulmonary edema. I'll be out of the hospital in a few days and the doctors recommend I carry an oxygen tank with me on the flight home." He was surprised that the airlines could require 48-hours notice in order to provide the FAA approved medical oxygen canister he needed. Although he experienced some delay, his travel agent and the airline carrier arranged for the medical oxygen he needed on board his homebound flight.*

Food on Board

Complimentary meals no longer are served routinely in coach class. On many airlines snacks may be sold to passengers, depending on your airline, and the length of the trip. Passengers in first class frequently receive complimentary snacks or a meal.

Personal Experience

SMA & BR: During a recent two-hour flight, Sue received a complimentary small packet of chips and a soft drink. Barbara, on her return non-stop flight from Hawaii to Minneapolis, received complimentary meals and complimentary soft drinks.

Because of the variation in food service between airlines and among scheduled flights, you should plan to bring enough food to cover the hours of your trip, especially if your medical condition is food dependent (i.e., diabetes, gluten sensitive).

Personal Experiences

SMA—A passenger became quite ill on an early flight. She explained that her motion sickness was aggravated by a lack of food. She had left home at four o'clock that morning and had not taken time to eat breakfast. Unaware that complimentary meals were no longer served regularly onboard the plane, she also had overlooked packing a snack for her early morning flight. She spent an uncomfortable two hours with only some ice chips and a glass of carbonated beverage to soothe her upset stomach.

Contact your airline several days before departure, and ask about your airline's food service policy. A few airlines may provide a hot sandwich or fresh cookies baked onboard. Others may offer meals prepared in a restaurant's kitchen and sold in-flight. Meal charges are estimated at $7-$15 per meal. Snack packs run approximately $5 (at this writing).

Arrival Procedures

Upon arrival at your destination, and before you leave the plane, remind the attendants if a wheelchair and a wheelchair attendant should be waiting for you.

Personal Experiences

SMA: Some of my best experiences at the airport have involved caring wheel-chair attendants. Our inbound flight connecting at O'Hare in Chicago was late so my husband and I arrived minutes after our scheduled outbound flight left the gate. Hurriedly, the gate attendant made arrangements for us to board another flight readying to pull away from its gate.

"It's the seventh gate on the left," he said. At the same time he signaled a wheelchair attendant who was in the area.

"I can walk," I told him.

"I'm sure you can." he smiled. "But that's why I'm here and I don't want you to miss another plane."

"But what about my husband," I asked.

"We'll just put him on the 'People Mover' over there," he laughed. "And don't worry, I'll keep track of him."

Yes, we made the plane. Thanks to our dedicated wheelchair attendant.

Do not leave the plane until someone arrives with a wheelchair for your use. Make certain the wheelchair attendant knows your destination in the terminal. This advice may seem unnecessary, but wheelchair attendants need to be reminded if you are going up or down stairs, for example. Ask them whether they can take you to another level of the terminal.

Personal Experiences

SMA: Recently, a friend told me about her 80-year-old mother's experience arriving at an airport. Her daughters, because of security regulations, could not enter the security zone to meet her at the boarding gate. Since the distance of the concourse was further than she should walk, she rode a motorized cart with multiple seats, available at most airport terminals. She told the driver she needed to go to baggage claim. He took her the long distance through her concourse, and stopped near the top of the escalator. He told her she should ride the escalator downstairs to baggage claim. Her arms full of packages, her coat and her tote bag in hand, she was uncertain whether she could keep her balance on the ride down the escalator. She later told her daughter, "I waited until some businessmen in suits came along and I stepped on the escalator behind them. I thought if I fell, one of them might catch me."

Motorized Wheelchairs or Scooters

Contact your carrier and ask their suggestion about the amount of time you should allow in preparing your powered wheelchair or scooter for storage aboard the plane. As we mention below, most carriers will suggest about two hours. You will need patience as you arrange for airline employees to place your powered wheelchair or scooter in the cargo bin.

Personal Experiences

SMA & BR: A friend of years past, who became a wheelchair-user following a spinal cord injury explained, "I've found I can do most things anyone else does. It just takes me a little longer." His sense of self-confidence was apparent as he described boarding a plane with his wheelchair.

Airlines recommend checking-in with your powered wheelchair or scooter at least 75 minutes to two hours prior to the scheduled departure. This time may vary among the airlines and terminals, requiring you to contact your airline for their suggestion. However, we suggest you allow at least two hours. Check-in lines and security lines require longer waiting periods today as security has become tighter and federal agents provide more thorough scrutiny. Do contact your airline for their specific recommendation for arrival time at the terminal.

Note: Even if you check-in less than one hour before flight time, the carrier will make a "reasonable effort" to accommodate your wheelchair. The airline, however, will not delay the flight in order to place your wheelchair or scooter on board.

Wheelchair Batteries
The battery on your wheelchair will be treated separately from the wheelchair, depending on the type battery you use.

Spillable Wet Cell Batteries
Sulfuric acid contained in wet cell batteries can, if spilled, corrode your wheelchair's wiring, frame, or parts of the aircraft. Most airlines refuse to carry a spillable battery unless it is removed and stored in a chemical-proof, spill-proof container. If the carrier removes the battery from

the wheelchair because of the DOT hazardous waste regulations, the carrier must provide packaging that meets safety requirements. Wheelchair batteries are packaged with no fee to the passenger.

Non-Spillable Dry Cell, Gel-Cell Batteries
Since 1995, nonspillable dry cell (gel-cell) batteries must be marked and identified as nonspillable, according to DOT rules. In addition, DOT hazardous materials regulations provide that it is unnecessary to remove a battery marked as nonspillable. If a battery is *not marked* as nonspillable, it can be removed from the wheelchair. During the loading and storing process, the battery must always be in an upright position.

Do Not Drain the Battery
A wheelchair battery may not be drained.

Packaging a Disconnected Battery
If DOT regulations require disconnecting the battery (because it contains hazardous materials); you can request packaging for the battery that meets safety requirements. Again, the carrier cannot charge you for such packaging.

Other Assistive Devices

Airline personnel now pay closer attention to canes, crutches and other assistive devises that might be used as weapons. You will be asked to store crutches and non-collapsible canes out of your reach, in the cabin's closet or below the cabin in the cargo areas of the plane. Keep your collapsible cane (such as a white cane) folded and placed in the overhead bin, or stored under the seat in your briefcase or large purse. You might need it in an emergency.

Current and Future Findings

Since the 9/11 Commission Report has been made public, you have no doubt experienced changes in security policies and practices at airline terminals and with airline carriers. And, there will be more to come.

Examples of proposed changes or those that already have been put into place include the following.

Prohibited Items

The Transportation Security Administration (TSA) categorizes the items prohibited from security checkpoints as "weapons, explosives, and incendiaries." Some items may seem harmless but may be used as a weapon.[2]

Checkpoint

Bringing prohibited items to a checkpoint without authorization could subject the passenger to criminal or civil prosecution. And, keep in mind that it is illegal to bring these items with you to a checkpoint even though it is done accidentally. Such items as cigarette lighters and butane lighters will be included in these categories. This list changes frequently, but you can update your information by going online to www.tsa.gov (Transportation Safety Administration). Several pages of "Permitted and Prohibited Items" provide extensive lists of items, clearly marked, as to whether they are permitted for Carry-on,

Checked or are *prohibited* altogether. The TSA also publishes a special section for "Travelers with Disabilities and Medical Conditions."

Kiosks

Kiosks, designed for passengers who need to mail home items that are banned onboard aircraft, have been installed in some of the large airport terminals. More are planned throughout the country. These kiosks offer automatic mailing and provide detailed instructions to passengers.

Food and Beverages

Many carriers offer an option of purchasing on board such items as snack boxes or sandwiches. Plans suggest that flights to Europe and business or first-class passengers will not be affected. You should, however, check with your airline. As an added precaution, carry a sandwich, fruit or other food items if your health requires it. The quality of water on airlines has come into question in recent times. Large airlines and the Environmental Protection Agency (EPA) are working together in an effort to remedy the situation. Even though it seems prudent to carry sealed bottled water with you, the 3-ounce limit applies.

Frequent Flyer Miles

Passengers purchasing tickets with frequent flyer miles earned by accumulating miles for past travel must be aware that some airlines tend to set aside fewer seats for these rewards than they have in the past. Many airlines offer these award miles (AAdvantage = American, Sky Miles = Delta,

Mileage Plus = United, World Perks = Northwest). Making your reservation early will help assure a seat in one of the special rewards seats. One airline has assured us that the bulkhead seats will continue to be available for passengers with a disability whether traveling as a Frequent Flyer or as a regularly ticketed passenger.

Changing Rules

Security and safety rules must be flexible and change as world events demand. For that reason, we recommend that you contact the Federal Aviation Administration (FAA) (online: www.faa.gov) and the Transportation Security Administration (TSA) (online: www.tsa.gov) or your airline regarding the latest requirements and recommendations. Enjoy a safe trip.

CHAPTER 4

ALL ABOARD:
Get on Track with Amtrak

The mention of Casey Jones, the Atchison, Topeka and Santa Fe line, the Empire Builder and the City of New Orleans bring fond memories to those of us who have ridden passenger trains or have dreamed of speeding through the prairie, the Rockies, or a quiet southern town on a moonlight night. Many people sense nostalgia upon simply hearing a distant train whistle. Amtrak still offers a pleasant journey to those persons who choose to travel the rails. Passengers with disabilities can find a number of services suited to them.

Personal Experience

SMA—My husband and I experienced a restful and scenic train trip along the banks of the Mississippi River and across the state of Wisconsin, arriving several hours later in Chicago.

We boarded the train at St. Paul, Minnesota during the early morning hours, and enjoyed both the ever-changing view from our coach seat and from the dining car's wide windows where we ate a leisurely breakfast.

I had reserved a wheelchair for the St. Paul and Chicago stations several weeks prior to our departure. The station agent told me he was noting my request on his computer (in fact, I watched him make the entry). Several wheelchairs were available at the St. Paul station upon our departure, but I saw only friends or family members pushing passengers the short distance to the train. Amtrak attendants did provide passengers the help they needed by rolling them across the metal boarding bridge and into the coach car. On the return trip, however, I noted an Amtrak attendant in Chicago assisting persons in wheelchairs during the much longer distance from the station to the coach car entrance.

Accessible Amtrak Stations

Contact your Amtrak Reservations Sales Assistant with questions about accessibility at their train stations. Call their toll free number 1-800-USA-RAIL (1-800-872-7245) or their TDD/TTY number 1-800-523-6590 and ask to be transferred to a Customer Service Agent if the Reservations Sales Assistant cannot answer your questions. Ask whether the stations you are using have staff on duty at the hour of your departure or arrival, and whether they have a high or low-level boarding platform.

The stations with Amtrak staff on duty usually will help wheelchair users move up and down steps and to and from the restrooms within the station. Passengers also may require boarding assistance. Stations with a high boarding platform use a metal bridge plate placed between the platform and passenger car. Low-level platforms can provide level boarding with "station-board" lifts. If you need assistance at these stations, notify Amtrak in advance. Lift requirements mandate an occupied wheelchair can weigh no more than 600 lbs./725kg.

Call Amtrak's toll-free number 1-800-USA-RAIL (1-800-872-7245) 24-hours prior to departure in order to request wheelchair-lift assistance, or about any other assistance relating to your disability. You will need to give them your reservation (confirmation) number or the credit card number to which you charged your ticket. Your reservation and your special needs will be forwarded to the appropriate station and train personnel.

Purchase Tickets

Once you have finalized your travel plans, make your reservation and buy your ticket as soon as possible. If you tell the ticket agent you need a short time to arrange to purchase your ticket, it may be held with a reservation for 24-hours or so before you must buy it. However, the agent's flexibility may depend on the number of seats that have been sold. Ticket agents also can help you determine the most convenient seating and the services you may need.

Personal Experiences

SMA—We purchased our tickets at the Amtrak station a few weeks before our trip. The ticket agent suggested we might want to reserve a Lower-Level (LL) seat since Rest Rooms as well as the entrance and exit door to the train were on that lower level. (Note: Lower Level seating is available only on trains that provide bi-level cars.) We found the Lower Level seating comfortable and convenient, providing ample legroom. Only twelve seats (six double seats) were available in our Lower Level unit, providing a traffic free, quiet atmosphere. Neither end of the Lower Level has doors opening to another car, so passengers cannot walk from one car to another, but must climb a narrow, enclosed stairway located in each Lower Level to reach the Upper Level. Upper Level units, with a power sliding door at either end of each car, allow passengers to walk from car to car, to the Dining car, the Club car or the Observation car. We caution you that the train sways from side to side as it speeds over the tracks. I found it possible, but not easy, to maintain good balance while walking the distance of the train while it was in motion. The dining car steward comes to each car, reserving the hour passengers want to dine (i.e., dinner at 5 p.m., 6 p.m., or 7 p.m.). We timed our meals in the dining car to coincide with the train's schedule (a copy should be available at your seat or from the train's attendant) so that we walked when the train stopped. Rather than making your way through the Upper Level of three or four cars, passengers with a mobility disability can stay in their seats, order from the menu and ask the train attendant to serve the food in their car. Or, you can bring food from home. Lower Level seating is reserved for passengers with disabilities, so designate your preferred seating when making reservations. Seats can sell out fast.

Charge To Your Credit Card

Amtrak accepts valid credit cards at the time you make your reservation online, by phone or at the ticket counter in the station. They will mail your ticket to you by U. S. Mail or you can pick it up at the station's ticket counter. Amtrak's online website (www.amtrak.com) also allows you to make your reservation and pay for your ticket by credit card. You must keep your Confirmation number in order to retrieve your ticket later at your station. Larger train stations (such as Chicago, Seattle, and Philadelphia) provide a Fast-Trak machine at the station where you pick-up your ticket by inserting your credit card through a narrow slit provided for that purpose. The online website will also provide graphic instructions for using the Fast-Trak machine, and explain how you can receive a printed boarding pass. If you prefer to have your ticket mailed to you by U.S. Mail, purchase your ticket at least one week before departure (again, you can use your credit card). You also can use their Toll-Free number or their TTY number in making your credit card payment.

If you cannot pay for your ticket in advance of boarding the train because of your disability and must pay for your ticket on the train, Amtrak will waive the extra charges usually assessed for this service. Keep in mind that the fares probably will increase as the passenger seats fill. Book early to receive your preference for accessible space and the best fare.

Amtrak is considering adjusting their ticket sales so that the busiest hours and the busiest lines are charged the highest fares. Conversely, making your reservation early and choosing off-peak hours should help provide you with lower fares.

Accessible Passenger Cars

At least one coach car, offering accessible seating and an accessible restroom, is available in every train. Open seating also may be available, permitting passengers to remain seated in their wheelchairs.

Personal Experiences

SMA—On our return trip from Chicago two double seats were removed from our car to make room for two wheelchair users. The train attendant came by periodically to check with them regarding their needs. She took their orders for food from the menu and served them in our car.

Accessible Bedrooms

One accessible bedroom is available in each sleeping car. At this writing, the bedrooms are available in two different designs, depending on the route you choose. Accessible bedrooms run the width of the train and allow room for one passenger with a wheelchair and one without a wheelchair. First Class fares for bedroom accommodations include meals that can be served in the dining car or your bedroom, depending on your mobility. The attendant is usually close by to help with housekeeping chores, such as turn-down service in the evening and putting the bed away again in the morning. Attendant call buttons are available in the bedroom and restroom areas.

Space and privacy in accessible bedrooms also provide an opportunity for passengers with limited mobility to change positions frequently since trips by rail can extend from several hours to several days.

Amtrak urges passengers with disabilities to follow these suggestions.

Available Equipment

Ask the reservation agent to describe the type of equipment Amtrak will use on your trip. Will the train include a dining car or a club car for sandwiches? Request information about the design of the bedrooms and other accessible space, as necessary.

Accessible Space

Seating space near accessible restrooms and in the Lower Level (where bi-level equipment is available) must be requested in advance. When assigned seating is not offered, Amtrak will try to provide for these requests on a first come basis. Whether traveling on a reserved or unreserved train, contact Amtrak in advance and reserve accessible space, a transfer seat and wheelchair space, according to your needs. Due to the limited number of bedrooms available, advance reservations are particularly important for passengers requiring accessible bedroom accommodations. Contact 1-800-YES-RAIL (1-800-872-7245); TDD/TTY: 1-800-523-6590.

Reserve Accessible Space

Reservations can be taken by phone or through the Amtrak web site. Accessible space should be reserved as early as possible. Reserved trains assign passengers to a certain car, but seating is often open (on a first come basis). Other trains are not reserved. This means general seating is on a first come basis for all passengers *except* those who need accessible space.

Personal Experiences

SMA—Because of the added legroom and the quiet atmosphere in the Lower Level, these seats are usually popular with able-bodied as well as passengers with disabilities. For that reason it is necessary to reserve a Lower Level seat (LL) as early as possible, telling the agent of your disability. The Conductor asked several passengers on our train to move to the Upper Level because they had no reservations in the Lower Level and told him they had no disability.

"Hold" Accessible Bedroom

Accessible bedroom accommodations will be held for persons with qualified mobility conditions up until 14 days before the train departs from its city of origin.

Accessible Seating in Club Cars

Amtrak offers accessible seating on *some* Club cars. Snacks and drinks are for sale on most trains, but you should ask about the variety of foods served in the Club Car (e.g., hot foods? cold foods? sandwiches?).

Carry-On And Checked Baggage

Use Amtrak's free identification tags to mark your baggage. You may carry-on two (2) pieces of baggage, if they are no more than 28"x22"x14". In addition you can carry-on such items as purses, laptops, and briefcases. A maximum of three pieces (maximum weight 50 pounds each) may be checked. Baggage weighing over 50 pounds will not be accepted as checked baggage. Amtrak security provides that only passengers with government issued picture identification can check baggage. When you pick-up your baggage, Amtrak will collect your claim check numbers. A storage fee will be charged for pieces left more than two days.

NOTE

Never check through your medications. Keep them with you since you will not be able to access your checked baggage from the time you leave your departure point until you arrive at your destination. On our return trip from Chicago, for example, one piece of my luggage did not arrive in Minneapolis. The Station staff person was informed and helpful about taking the proper steps to alert personnel to the description of my luggage. Two days later the Station agent phoned me to say my luggage would arrive that night. We found no missing clothing and the luggage was intact.

Railway Discount Fares

Amtrak offers rail fare discounts for senior passengers, passengers with disabilities and other specific passengers. Amtrak notes you must present written documentation of your disability at the ticket counter. Passengers also must present written documents when boarding the train, in one of the following forms:

- A letter from your doctor
- Proof of membership in a disability organization such as The American Foundation for the Blind
- An identification card, such as those used by numerous transit systems, such as Paratransit

No Double Dipping

Amtrak does not allow passengers to take advantage of two different passenger discounts. A senior with a disability, for example, cannot use a discount for both a disability and for senior status.

No Smoking

Amtrak trains no longer allow smoking in any part of the train. Conductors (at their discretion) may announce a smoking break at certain stops where passengers are permitted a short smoke break while standing on the station platform outside the train. Two sounds from the engine's horn signal that passengers must return immediately to the train.

Travel with Your Service Animal

Service animals must be *trained* as service animals, and can accompany you free of charge in all passenger areas, including stations, trains, and Amtrak Thruway motorcoaches. When you make your reservation, inform the Amtrak agent that you will be bringing your Service animal with you. You must keep your animal under control at all times. Animals causing a disturbance can be turned over to local animal control officials. When you board the train, tell the Conductor that you will need to walk your animal at station stops. You must remain close to the train and preboard promptly at the Conductor's signal (listen for two sounds from the engine's horn).

Food Service

Amtrak offers snacks in their Club car and meal service from their Dining car. Most trains provide some food service although the cost is not included in regular coach fare. Meal service may be ordered from the menu and served in your room, at your seat, in the lounge car or in the dining car, when certain conditions allow. Special diets such as kosher, vegetarian, and vegan may be available on your route with 72-hours advance notice. Contact Customer Service for information about special diets and food service on your train. To reserve your meal, call 1-800-872-7245 or TTY Service at 1-800-523-6590. Because delays may be unavoidable, Amtrak suggests that you carry food to meet your dietary needs (diabetes, for example). Amtrak will provide ice for storing insulin in your cooler if you give advance notice.

Security Rules—Passengers must provide government issued photo Identification. We suggest you keep your identification on your person at all times. Amtrak accepts photo driver's license, photo ID for non-drivers, a Passport, or a university, college or high school photo ID. Passengers under 18-years-of-age should have their ID available if they wish to purchase items. Certain items cannot be carried onboard with you, such as:

- firearms, guns, ammunition
- large sharp objects such as ice picks and swords
- liquid bleach, tear gas, corrosive chemicals

Security policies change frequently. Contact Amtrak prior to your next trip and ask for current information about security measures on their trains. You also can visit the Amtrak website at www.amtrak.com for specific safety requirements or phone Amtrak's Customer Service toll free number.

Personal Experience

SMA—We observed variations in security policies from one station to another. I did not have my ID with me prior to boarding the train in Minneapolis-St. Paul. The station agent assured us we would have no problem. We checked baggage, passed by the Conductor and found our assigned seats with no questions asked. On the re-

turn trip, however, the agent in Chicago refused to allow me to check baggage until my husband arrived with his ticket and picture identification.

Another train in the Pennsylvania-Newark Corridor was stopped mid-route and passengers' identifications were inspected. The train was delayed for about ninety minutes. Just another reminder that you should take along extra food or medication in your carry-on if your health requires that protection.

Medical Oxygen

If you need medical oxygen on your trip, inform the Amtrak reservation agent that you are bringing oxygen onboard with you. Secure your oxygen tanks on board so they will not fall and cannot move about freely, striking another object. Detach any wheels that may be fastened to the tanks while on board the train. If you need on-board electrical power for your equipment, you cannot rely solely on the train to provide electrical power. (See www.amtrak.com for additional details about Equipment Requirements or contact 1-800-872-7245 or TDD/TTY 1-800-523-6590.).Oxygen cannot be used in or near smoking areas. You may not carry an oxygen tank with you when passing through a smoking area. Calculate your travel time from boarding until you arrive at your destination. Amtrak suggests you "bring at least 20 percent additional oxygen to cover possible delays or disruptions."

Personal Experience

SMA—When planning a trip on Amtrak, we've found that we need to consider a few issues that are spe-

cific to the trains. First, you must build-in extra time for your trip. The trip from St. Paul to Chicago, for example, requires at least eight to nine hours. Unexpected stops do occur, so you should plan for some delay. One of our trains stopped for two separate medical emergencies. One passenger became ill and was taken to the nearest hospital. Because all cars are Non-Smoking, the train also stopped at several stations for ten minute smoking breaks. We ran an hour late on our trip to Chicago and thirty minutes late getting into St. Paul on the return trip.

Our train bound for Chicago in December arrived six hours late in Minneapolis, after making its way across the country from Seattle. We kept up-to-date with their schedule by going to the Online Home page (www.amtrak.com). The "train status" panel on the Home page will give you the current location and time of your scheduled train. We were able to stay at home for four hours before heading off to the train terminal by using the Internet. You can also reach Amtrak at 1-800-YES-RAIL (1-800-872-7245). Passengers who had boarded on the West Coast visited with us in the Dining Car and told us Amtrak scheduled meetings with passengers who were missing their connections in Chicago. These passengers were given options as for how they could best reach their destinations out of Chicago.

Second, assess your willingness and your patience to spend eight or more hours (whatever the length of your trip) with passengers chosen at random. We found our traveling companions helpful and interesting, representing a broad mix of Americana. In addition to the Club

Car and Dining Car, some trains include an Observation Car. Seats swivel offering a view of the scenery surrounding you. TV or a movie (on some trains) may be an option for your entertainment. The Dining Car offers tables for four people. If your party is less than four, the Amtrak dining car steward determines where you sit and your dining partners. We have enjoyed the passengers we have met. A Semi-truck driver traveling back to the east coast to pick up a new truck and his next load, for example, shared many interesting stories about his life on the road. We were dinner companions with a church organist and, coincidentally, a classical soprano soloist who performs with a national company. She was traveling from her home in New York to her parents' home in North Dakota. We also visited with an eighty-year-old grandmother who sat across the aisle from us. She insisted on snapping our photo with her digital camera, as she reached her destination.

You can ignore your traveling companions or you can become engaged. The choice is yours. But it is a factor to consider before you purchase your tickets.

For further information, phone Amtrak or check out their online website (www.amtrak.com).

CHAPTER 5

TRAVELING BY MOTOR COACH

More passengers board Greyhound and other scheduled independent regional bus lines than ever before. Whether exploring the country, going to work, scheduling a shopping excursion or visiting friends and relatives, passengers with disabilities can find motor coaches and van lines a convenient and reasonably priced means of travel.

We have chosen Greyhound as our model because it is the only bus line operating throughout the United States providing consistent rules and policies for travelers with disabilities. Regional and local lines operate under policies, rules and schedules that vary from area to area. Check with your local line for any questions about reservations, seat assignments, transporting assistive devices and other issues related to your disability.

Speaking of Greyhound

Beginning in 2004, Greyhound cut a number of their routes, eliminating over 200 bus stops throughout the West and Middle Western United States. However, regional private bus lines and van lines have begun picking up passengers at some cities and smaller towns once serviced by Greyhound. In fact, both riders and the smaller lines may find the new arrangement beneficial. Ask your travel agent where you can find the nearest public intrastate or interstate bus terminals.

Greyhound provides full service at their larger bus terminals, ranging from ticketing to services for persons with disabilities. Some Greyhound bus stops, marked with a large [B], only offer service for passengers, and do not *handle baggage or sell tickets.*

No Reservations Policy

Greyhound follows a procedure that is different than most airlines and rail lines. You will find, for example, that Greyhound's no-reservation policy seats passengers on a first come first served basis. They place no limit on the number of tickets they can issue. When a bus sells out all seats, they may "call-up" another bus (referred to as an extra section). Adding an extra section depends, however, on the availability of an extra bus.

Ticketing

Although you do not need a reservation, ticketing is easily transacted through a variety of options.

"Will Call"

In some cities you can order tickets online and pick them up at the bus terminal before boarding. "Will Call" tickets can be ordered through the Internet and paid for with your credit card. You must, however, present your credit card, the reference number (as shown following the purchase on your computer screen) and a photo ID at the time you pick-up your ticket. If you do not present your credit card at the counter, a fee will be charged. If you pick up the ticket, but are not the credit card holder, you must present your reference number and your picture ID. Rules can change quickly, so check with Greyhound's toll free number 1-800-231-2222 (USA only) for additional information.

Tickets by Mail
Tickets may be purchased online and delivered to you at your U.S. Mail postal address. They must be ordered at least 10 mailing days in advance and paid for with a valid credit card issued by a U.S. Bank. You may want to ask about the non-refundable fee for this service.

Tickets at the Greyhound Agency
Tickets are available for purchase at the terminal's ticket counter or at a Greyhound Agency. However, you should arrive at least an hour before your departure if you plan to buy your ticket at the terminal.

Tickets by phone
Phone the Greyhound Toll-free number (USA only) at 1-800-231-2222. You may purchase your ticket with your credit card.

Discounted fares
These tickets are usually non-refundable and must be purchased at least 7 days in advance. Some restrictions may apply. For example, certain holidays may not be included at the discounted prices. Check with Greyhound for further information. You can phone the Fare and Schedule Telephone Center at 1-800-229-9424.

Greyhound Disabilities Assist Line

When you make plans for your trip with Greyhound Bus Lines, travelers with disabilities should contact the Greyhound Disabilities Assist Line 1-800-752-4841 to inform their personnel about your special needs. According to Greyhound, one of their representatives will discuss your special needs and will store this data in Greyhound's databank. Your request will allow them an opportunity to provide the equipment and information to the personnel who will be assisting you. They also ask you to remind the Greyhound employees (or Greyhound's contractors) at each location along your route that you have special needs. Remind them about the specific help you have requested. Do you have mobility needs? food dependent needs (such as diabetes)? hearing or vision needs? They can respond quicker and answer your questions in a timely manner if you talk with them directly.

Accessible Equipment

Some, but not all, coaches in Greyhound's fleet are accessible. In other words, these coaches offer an accessible lavatory and/or a wheelchair lift. If you need an accessible coach, you must give the Greyhound Disabilities Assist Line advance notice. Contact them at least 48-hours, but not more that seven days in advance of your departure. They require at least 48-hours to transfer their accessible coaches to your requested location. If you do not provide 48-hours prior notice, Greyhound will attempt to assist you, but will not delay their departure if an accessible coach is not available.

Guidelines for Traveling on Greyhound

Passengers informed about the following guidelines can enjoy a safer, more fulfilling bus trip.

Arrive and Check-in Early

Greyhound will require a photo identification card (use your government issued driver's license, non-driver's identification card or passport) when you check in at the terminal's ticket window. Passengers with disabilities must arrive at the terminal at least one hour prior to departure. You will need time to purchase a ticket (if you have not pre-purchased it), check baggage and locate the departure gate. Boarding generally occurs 15 to 30 minutes prior to the bus leaving the terminal. Although this is the current suggested time schedule, you should contact Greyhound a few days prior to departure in the event of changes.

Assist Passengers Boarding

Providing Greyhound employees (and their contractors) 48-hours notice will give them the time they need to help you with boarding and deboarding, with baggage, transfers and stowing and retrieving your mobility devices. Even though you have notified the *Greyhound Disabilities Assist Line,* you must remind each driver about your special needs, so they can be available to help you at rest stops, meal stops and at transfer points.

Assistive Devices

Mobility aids that fit the space can be stowed in the overhead compartment provided they can be stowed safely. Otherwise, they will be placed in the baggage compartment located beneath and outside the bus. The baggage compartment is 33-inches x 33-inches x 48-inches. Mobility aids cannot exceed 200 pounds. Allow time for loading and unloading your aids and avoid delays for yourself and other passengers.

Checked and Carry-On

Each adult passenger is allowed two pieces of *checked baggage free,* and each child is allowed one piece free. Children under 2-years of age have no baggage allowance.

Each piece must weigh no more than 50 pounds, and passengers can expect an extra charge of $20-$30 (based on distance traveled) for each overweight piece.

Two pieces of *carry-on baggage* are permitted each customer, and must fit under the seat or in the overhead bin. Greyhound will not accept plastic or paper bags as checked baggage and recommends the use of shipping containers available in many terminals for a reasonable fee.

Rules change from time to time so we suggest you contact the bus company about their *current* allowable number of pieces of luggage, dimensions and weight for each item of baggage.

Baggage

Baggage must be marked with an identification tag stating your name, address and telephone number. ID tags are available at the customer counter. *Do not check your prescription medication. All medications should be carried with you in your carry-on bag.* Checked baggage will not be available to you until you arrive at your destination. Greyhound will not allow your Laptop computer as checked baggage, but you can carry it on as one of the two pieces of baggage you are allowed.

Questions and Prohibited Items

Contact Greyhound for their *Prohibited Items List* of items you cannot check or carry-on. If you have questions about Greyhound's policies regarding baggage, you can find their website at www.greyhound.com. Look for the section on Travel Information: Customers with Disabilities. You also can phone the Greyhound Disabilities Assist Line 1-800-752-4841.

Medical Information

Carry your medical information (name, address, phone number, your doctor's name and phone number, your pharmacy's name and phone number and a list of your medicines) on your person at all times. Carry your medications in carry-on bags. Baggage you have checked through will be placed in the baggage compartment located beneath and on the outside of the bus. These items will not be available to you until you reach your destination. Bring along your health insurance identification card (Medicare, Blue Cross/Blue Shield or other insurance carrier).

Medical Oxygen

Passengers are allowed to carry up to four canisters of medical oxygen with them. Two (2) canisters can be placed inside the coach. Two (2) additional canisters must be placed in the baggage compartment in protective cases and with safety caps on the valves. For further details contact Greyhound Disabilities Assist Line 1-800-752-4841.

No Smoking
All coaches are designated "No Smoking" in compliance with Federal Regulations. Greyhound also enforces a no drug, no alcohol policy.

Personal Identification
Carry with you a government issued picture I.D. such as your driver's license or passport. If you are 18 years of age and older, keep your driver's license or other government issued photo I.D. available for ticket agents or security guards.

Priority Seating
Priority seating is available and means the "first row directly behind and across from the driver." The "wheelchair securement areas" also are designated as priority seating. If those seats are taken, passenger(s) sitting in those seats may be asked to move to another seat, but cannot be required to move. Questions? Contact Greyhound Disabilities Assist Line 1-800-752- 4841.

Proof-of-Disability
Proof-of-disability is not required by Greyhound.

Personal Care Attendant (PCA)
Greyhound invites you to travel on your own with Greyhound provided you do not need help with personal services, such as eating or using the Rest Room. If you need a Personal Care Attendant (PCA), Greyhound may provide a one-way ticket at a 50-percent discount for the PCA who travels with you. Greyhound will assist you at their Greyhound Disabilities Assist Line 1-800-752- 4841. An

outline of this program's guidelines is also available online at www.greyhound.com.

Sample Guidelines for PCA Program

- Customer must request approval for participation in the PCA program and submit his/her PCA's name when making a reservation. Participation will depend on the assistance requested by the customer, not on the customer's disability.

- PCA must submit a picture ID before Greyhound issues the ticket.

- PCA must be at least 12 years old and must provide the service the Customer needs.

- Customer must request a PCA ticket 24-hours prior to departure time. If the Customer is requesting a bus with wheelchair lift equipment, the request for the PCA's ticket must be made 48-hours prior to departure.

- Customer and PCA must travel the entire trip together.

Other rules apply and can be found online at www.greyhound.com or by phoning the Greyhound Disabilities Assist Line 1-800-752-4841. You can expect to hear recorded messages before you are asked to continue to an agent. In our experience, the Greyhound Assist Line has responded quickly and with detailed, useful information. We have been treated courteously and have felt we were not rushed with our question or their answer.

Personal Experience

BR—Several years ago, I traveled by Greyhound Bus to Chicago to attend a friend's graduation from seminary. Another friend accompanied me, serving as my sighted guide (at that time Greyhound paid her fare both ways). We needed to provide proof of my blindness and to notify the company several days prior to departure that I would have a sighted-guide traveling with me.

The trip was flawless. The rest stops along the way were negotiated without incident. The seats were comfortable and the driver courteous and helpful. While riding the bus is time-consuming, it is an enjoyable way to travel if one has the time. Planning ahead made the trip even more enjoyable.

Trained Service Animals

Only *trained* service animals can travel with passengers with a disability. It's important to bring along official proof that your animal is trained for that purpose. Your animal must ride in your passenger's space and may not sit or stand in the aisle nor sit in a seat. You must keep your animal under control (by leash, harness, or carrier, for example) at all times.

Travel with a Minor

A minor, traveling with an adult Personal Care Attendant (PCA), will be charged a full adult fare. Inquiries about travel restrictions for minors with disabilities can be directed to Greyhound Customers with Disabilities Assist Line 1-800-752-4841.

Food Service and Greyhound

Greyhound Bus Lines schedule stops at their Greyhound Food Service restaurants where passengers can purchase sandwiches or other snacks. Passengers usually will be allowed several minutes to visit the shop and purchase food, a magazine, and other sundries, as desired. Buses try to maintain their scheduled routes and their arrival and departure times. Weather and mechanical problems, however, can cause unexpected delays. Confirm your schedule before you board. Diabetics and other passengers whose health requires food at certain times should bring enough carry-on food and medication to cover unexpected delays and unscheduled stops. Also, carry snacks such as candy, orange juice or fresh fruit in case of an emergency.

Submit Your Complaints

If you wish to file a complaint relating to violation of your rights under the Americans with Disabilities Act (ADA), phone 1-800-755-2357 as soon as possible or send a written statement to:

Greyhound Lines, Inc.
ADA Compliance Office
P.O. Box 660362
Dallas, Texas 75266-0362

CHAPTER 6

GET SMARTER WHEN YOU CHARTER

Many passengers with disabilities, who travel by bus, choose interstate commercial buses such as Greyhound. There are, however, social organizations, professional organizations and other groups who charter buses for travel to states throughout the country or within their own states. They enjoy traveling together and participating in activities such as church meetings, leisure outings, political activities and senior events. Passengers place trust in the church, club, or other organization that engages a bus company and driver to provide safe transportation.

Personal Experience

SMA—When our church organized a trip to Iowa for some of its members, I enthusiastically joined the group. Our music director had scheduled a day with the designer and manufacturer of the church's new pipe organ. The music director also made arrangements for leasing a bus and none of us checked further details about the charter contract. Why should we? Our music direc-

tor paid close attention to detail. We trusted him, our vestry and our rector. As it turned out, we enjoyed an exciting day looking at the plans for our new organ and listening to the details of the many standards a pipe organ must meet. We arrived home safely later that day.

The trip I described might have turned out differently. Most of us have heard or read reports of chartered buses rolling down an embankment, colliding with other motor vehicles, or swerving off the road. Investigations later may identify faulty brakes, driver error, inadequate maintenance, rain slick highways or other causes for the mishap.

The Federal Motor Carrier Safety Administration (FMCSA), as part of the U.S. Department of Transportation (DOT), makes every effort to provide safe transportation for all motor coach passengers. Their scope is broad, extending minimum safety standards to include the bus companies and the buses they operate as well as overseeing the physical qualifications and the operating rules drivers must follow. Their intent covers both the regularly scheduled bus lines such as Greyhound, and chartered buses that offer transportation to special groups.

The Bus, Van or Other Vehicle

Inquire about vehicle standards, including:

- What is the size of the company's fleet? How frequently is each bus or van used? You are trying to determine whether the company keeps an adequate number of buses and vans so their fleet can be regularly rotated for servicing.

- How frequently do the vehicles undergo periodic inspections?
- What restrictions, if any, apply to each of their vehicles?

The Company

To protect your group, the Federal Motor Carrier Safety Administration (FMCSA) suggests that the person in charge of arranging for the chartered bus inquire about the safety practices of the chartered motor coach company *before* contracting with them. The person in charge of your group should ask the Motor Coach Company about the following:

- How long has the company been in the business of chartering buses? In other words do they have a track record of caring for their equipment properly? Do they show a consistently good safety record?
- What is the company's DOT number? Your group can use the DOT number to check the carrier's safety rating.

The Driver

Charter only from a company who *enforces* a drug-free, alcohol-free work environment among their drivers. Then ask for the following:

- Does the driver qualify under DOT regulations?
- List the date the driver was last licensed, the driver's medical certification, and any limitations the license carries for the driver.

Insurance

What dollar amount of public liability insurance does the charter company carry? The person responsible should ask for (and receive) proof of financial responsibility before signing a contract with the Charter Company.

Insurance Coverage

Call the Federal Motor Carrier Safety Administration (202) 358-7000 (this is *not* a toll free number) in order to receive information about a carrier's insurance coverage.

References

Ask for references from groups similar to your own (church groups, senior citizen groups, etc). Look for other bus companies if a company will not provide references.

Safety Rating

Call the U.S. Department of Transportation (DOT) at (703) 280-4001 (this is *not* a toll free number) for information about a carrier's safety rating.

Special Needs for Travelers with Disabilities

Ask the carrier or contracting company the following:

- How do they provide for the special needs of persons with disabilities?
- Are their coaches equipped with wheelchair lifts?
- Are their coaches equipped with accessible bathrooms?
- Do they provide assistance for persons with disabilities who are getting off and on the bus?

- Do their buses accept service animals onboard their coaches?
- Do they charge a fee for a service animal?
- Do their buses make rest stops so passengers can buy snacks, meals and walk about?

Personal Experience

SMA—My friend belongs to an organization that sponsors an annual trip for the Senior Citizens in their group. They have chartered buses in the state of Indiana and traveled to Branson, Missouri, Nashville, Tennessee, the state of Ohio, and other places of interest. They usually plan a two-night stay. Since senior citizens may have special needs, their group has made a point of using a chartered bus equipped to accommodate travelers with disabilities. The bus offers a boarding lift for any member who uses a wheelchair. The driver assists the passenger(s) who need to wheel onto the lift and temporarily buckle onto the lift until rolled into the bus. These buses usually provide grab bars in the rest room areas also. Their group has found they need to schedule the bus from six-months to one year in advance of their trip.

Subcontracting Agreements

Will the contracting company who contracts directly with your group subcontract to (use) another motor carrier's equipment and/or driver on the trip (during all or any part of the trip)? If so, your group must receive information about the equipment to be used and the driver assigned to your trip.

These suggestions are for the safety and protection of you and the members of your group who charter a bus. Responsible companies can and will immediately give you answers or help you find the answers to the questions we've proposed or to any other questions that may be of concern to your group.

Enjoy your trip!

CHAPTER 7

TAKE A BRAKE

Traveling by car offers several advantages to traveling by plane, train or bus. First, one can travel on one's own schedule. Second, traveling by car can be an economical way to take a trip. Third, one can spend as much time at a chosen location as one wants. Traveling by car makes one a wanderer, an explorer, and a geographic detective. This section is devoted to taking a trip when you yourself are the driver or when you are a carefree passenger simply enjoying the sights.

Many people with disabilities have drivers' licenses. Cars can be adapted with hand controls. Vans can be equipped with a lift. Driving courses are available for persons with disabilities at most rehabilitation centers or centers for independent living. Just as drivers' licenses indicate the need for one to wear glasses, your disability and its restrictions may be listed on your driver's license. Many states also issue stickers or license plates which indicate that one is disabled and, therefore, entitled to handicap parking. You may want to check with your local Motor Vehicle Department or your state council on disability before leaving home. If you are looking for a specific Center for Independent Living, check the internet at www.virtualcil.net/cil/ for the list of independent living centers throughout the country. Click on the colorful map (choose the state you plan to visit) or click on the text offered as a list of states below the map. These centers can offer you invaluable information about local resources. For example, if your wheelchair needs repair, or if your van or car needs additional adaptive equipment or repairs, or if you are looking for accessible hotels, local centers for independent living can assist you. In addition, oftentimes, these centers are staffed by people with disabilities whose experience in that town or city is first hand.

The Internet can also assist you in finding local dialysis centers while you are traveling. Reserve time beforehand with that center to ensure you will be serviced quickly and effectively. Much of the information offered in the other sections of this book apply to your travel by car. In short, plan ahead.

Many cities (and states) offer "access guides," which can acquaint you with the accessible sights and available events. People with disabilities are entitled to discount entrance fees to national parks and monuments. Numerous travel agencies specialize in planning trips for persons with disabilities. Even if you do not need your trip planned by such an agency, they may be able to help you with city brochures or discount fees to various events or sites. Check the internet or a library for assistance in finding one of these travel agencies.

The Chamber of Commerce or the Visitors Bureau in the cities you wish to visit can also assist you. This is an excellent time to be a person with a disability who wants to travel. Awareness about the need for accessibility has spread to most businesses that depend on tourist dollars. People with disabilities have become desirable guests who are welcomed graciously.

Include a Styrofoam cooler when planning your trip. Insulin users can use the cooler to keep insulin cool. Those travelers dependent on regular meals will have food, even if you do not find an accessible restaurant on time. A supply of potable water can also be carried.

Being a strong advocate on your own behalf is especially important when traveling by car. Laws which protect persons with disabilities strictly regulate airlines, buses, and trains. When traveling by car, you are still protected by The Americans with Disabilities Act, but you will need to be very clear in articulating what you need. Do not accept a room with a bathroom too small to enter with your wheelchair. Managers of hotels, parks, and restaurants are usually friendly and helpful. They cannot read your mind, however, or know your specific needs unless you articulate them. Your enjoyment will be enhanced when you are willing to ask for what you want and when you are persistent until your needs are met.

Personal Experience

BR—On a recent trip to Hawaii, I chose not to go down to the beach. The walk was long and steep and I had been told that there were no benches on which to sit when I got there. The trolley which ought to have been available was out of order. I was given incorrect information, and because I was not persistent, I missed the reef, the sand and the waves. Next time, I will follow my own advice.

Don't let the fears of others circumscribe your adventure. You are the best judge of what you *want* to do as well as what you *can* do. Be appropriately careful without being overly cautious. Plan carefully and then remain open to unplanned possibilities. Don't miss the adventure of a lifetime. It just may be around the next corner.

CHAPTER 8

PUTTING IT ALL TOGETHER!

Attention to small details can become not only important, but also necessary to our well being when organizing a travel itinerary. The excitement of visiting new and interesting places often overwhelms our focus for preventing troublesome health issues. Whatever our mode of transportation, we should be prepared for a few challenges along the way. With that in mind, this chapter is designed to help minimize or prevent such glitches.

Although many tips in this chapter are new, some not-to-be-overlooked ideas are reminders from earlier chapters. A checklist is provided for your use at the end of this chapter.

Juggling Your Way Through the Terminal

Moving through a terminal, whether airline, bus line, or rail line, travelers often feel they are assuming the role of a juggler or a tight wire artist trying to balance brief case, baggage, tickets and various personal items. Most passengers just hope to make their way through the terminal with their belongings intact. Dealing with baggage check-in, security check points and ticket kiosks can test the physical stamina and patience of even the most experienced traveler. Passengers with disabilities handle the same items able-bodied passengers carry. In addition they may travel with a cane, crutches, a service animal, personal oxygen tank or wheelchair. Most of us try to reduce the tension that occurs under the strain of travel.

> *Personal Experience*
>
> *SMA—My husband and I live with cardiovascular disease and have learned that certain situations such as rushing to make deadlines produce excessive stress. In our state of health we want to avoid symptoms such as shortness of breath. We plan for each step along the route and allow extra time so we can remain as unruffled as possible. If our schedule looks tight, we reserve a wheelchair at the time we book our tickets. In our situation, we book online or by phone. We arrive early at the terminal and enjoy a glass of water or juice, and my husband reads the newspaper while we wait. During a stopover in the Atlanta airport terminal, we were rushing to catch our connecting flight. The wheelchair attendant was waiting with two wheelchairs as we had requested. She wisely suggested we use the faster multiple-seat motorized (golf cart type) transport. Thanks to her advice, we easily covered the distance to our connecting gate with time to spare.*

Packing Light

Several days before departure, list the necessary items you will take along. The nice-to-have-with-you, but unnecessary items can be laid aside until you're *certain* you have space in your baggage. This is best done when you feel unhurried and can concentrate on putting together the things you *must* have with you on your trip. Carriers have become strict about limiting the number of bags as well as the weight of both carry-on and checked baggage charging significant fees for overweight baggage. Check with your carrier for the most recent baggage requirements. Airlines apply strict rules about carry-on baggage, so you must check with your carrier and the Transportation Security Administration's website www.tsa.gov for a current list of items that can and cannot be carried onboard the plane.

Most carriers place signs near the baggage check-in area or hand out brochures to make certain passengers understand their baggage limitations. Amtrak usually leaves a recorded phone message on your home phone as a reminder. Greyhound, and other bus lines, may have their baggage requirements online (www.greyhound.com). Or, phone the Customers with Disabilities Travel Assistance Line at 1-800-752-4841 for their guidelines on baggage and any other equipment you may need with you on your trip. The following suggestions can help reduce the weight, volume and number of pieces you carry. No doubt you can add to this list.

Baggage

It's easy to overlook the weight of an empty piece of baggage. You can determine the weight of your empty pieces of baggage by asking the baggage department at your favorite shop, or checking online for the specific brand you own or wish to purchase. You can also weigh each piece on a bathroom scale by weighing yourself with the baggage in your hand, then stepping off the scale, weighing yourself without the baggage and subtracting the difference. Some luggage companies have made efforts to manufacture their brands in lighter and more efficient designs by molding their pieces from light weight, sturdy materials. They also eliminate overall lining, replacing it with two or three cloth pockets attached with Velcro. If you're buying new luggage, it's worthwhile checking the weight. You may be surprised at the differences. Don't assume that soft-side luggage is lighter weight.

Personal Experience

SMA—On a flight to Los Angeles (LAX), my husband and I used identical luggage and each packed in our own style. That is, I tried to be aware of packing efficiently and lightweight, and he took what he thought he might need. When the airline weighed our individual pieces of luggage, mine weighed in at 38.5 pounds and his at 48.8. Mine was 11.5 pounds below the fifty-pound limit and his was 1.2 pounds below the limit. We've included this as both an example of packing prudently and also demonstrating the value of carrying the new lighter weight luggage. Every tenth of a pound can make a difference.

Shoes

Will you really need two pair of athletic shoes, three pair of black casual shoes and two pair of dress shoes to round out your social and business life while you're traveling? Adding two extra pair of shoes may cause your baggage to be over the required weight. Shoes can be bulky and heavy and must be comfortable. If you need special shoes or braces made to accommodate your special needs, check with your carrier for their packing suggestions. Some special equipment may not count toward your maximum weight limit.

Heavy coat or jacket
Can you wear, rather than pack, your suit jacket or coat (depending on the season)? Thoughtfully assess your clothing, considering the weather and your needs.

Books or recorded books
Reading is relaxing for travelers and a good time to catch up on those books you've been waiting to read. Shop your local bookstores (used and new) for lightweight paperbacks rather than the hard covers. Paperbacks are lighter and less expensive, especially used ones. Recorded books and magazines are alternatives for those of us whose disability affects our vision. A portable lightweight audio-cassette or CD player is convenient for books, magazines and music. The I-pod is a current favorite that allows music or books to be downloaded through your computer. Those who use cassettes or CDs may also consider bringing mailer(s) that fold flat and are available through the United States Post Office. Pre-addressed padded envelopes also serve the same purpose. Returning cassettes or CDs as you travel is an efficient way to leave room for new items you purchase along the way. The National Library Service for the Blind and Physically Handicapped, a nationwide free service for persons with disabilities, provides a plastic box with an addressed label and postage included for free return mailing. Their

recordings are presently on 4-track cassette tapes, and they loan clients a 4-track cassette player free-of-charge. A smaller hand-held 4-track player, suitable for travel, also can be purchased. When traveling by car, standard cassettes sometimes called "talking books" are available for rent at some restaurants. Cracker Barrel Restaurants, for example, allow you to rent cassettes at one of their many restaurants and return it to another Cracker Barrel location along your route.

Medicines and Medical Equipment

Organize your medications and medically related items such as assistive devices. Stowing canes, crutches, oxygen tanks and wheelchairs require planning. If you travel with a collapsible white cane, you will not be asked to store it, and will be allowed to keep it in your purse or briefcase where it is available to you. Make certain the storage space your car, bus, plane or train provides adequately meets your needs for these devices. Can these items be stowed in the passenger section (of your bus, plane or train) or must they go into the cargo hold (baggage area)? If you're unsure, call your carrier. You also need to plan where such items can be stowed in your car or van. Commonly, packing at the last minute causes passengers to become frustrated and disorganized, overlooking items that will be sorely needed during the trip.

Documenting your health

Passengers with disabilities should be ready to provide medical information to their carrier's crew in case of a medical emergency. You may want to use plastic covers or bags to protect these documents. Consider organizing your official documents around these three areas: 1. Personal Identification Documents; 2. Medical Documents; and 3. Insurance Documents. Use the following lists to check-off items as you pack.

1. Personal identification documents

- Driver's license, or non-driver's identification (current)
- Luggage tags with your name, address and phone number
- Luggage tags on the inside and outside of your luggage.
- Passport, if necessary
- Tickets with your name, accurate dates, hours of arrival/departure and destination
- Social security card
- Credit card, if you purchased your ticket with the credit card and/or you plan to use it on your trip

2. Electronic devices

Electronic devices also provide a great deal of personal information about you. Protect cell phones, laptops, and handheld units that can be left behind in airplane seats, cabs, rental cars, train seats, bus seats or on shuttle buses. Mark your name and the appropriate contact information on these electronic devices so that you can be contacted for their safe return.

A Word of Caution to Passengers with a Pacemaker/ Defibrillator. Discuss with your physician any risk you may encounter in passing through metal detectors. You may wish to request a pat-down as an option for your security check.

3. Medical documents

Passengers with disabilities need to carry with them documents that provide information about their health. All information must be current. Particularly, check your prescriptions. Keep the following information in your purse or briefcase.

- Medical prescriptions for medicines, test tapes (if you are diabetic and test your blood glucose), and other supplies requiring a prescription.
- Your physician's business card or his/her name, address, and phone number (handwritten or typed) in your wallet. Many of us look to one physician as our primary care physician or family doctor, but may also want to include the name and office number of certain specialists. Travelers with disabilities may want to include, for example, their neurologist, ophthalmologist, or any specialist who treats them regularly.
- Your pharmacy's business card or address and phone number (handwritten or typed).

- Prescriptions for eyeglasses or contact lens in case of loss or breakage.
- Medications. Pack medications in 1-quart size, clear plastic sealable bags. All medication should be in your carry-on baggage. Using clear plastic bags facilitates passing through security check-points. Make certain you know where your medications are at all times. Do not check through with your baggage.

4. Insurance documents

Include accident, automobile, hospital, Medicare, Medicaid, physician, supplemental and most coverage you carry. These usually include an identification card (the size of your driver's license) that can be carried in your wallet. It's also important that you know where to locate your policy and that you leave such information with your relative, lawyer or friend where they can find them in an emergency.

- *Medical insurance cards.* Memorize your social security and Medicare identification numbers, if possible.
- Make certain your *health insurance policies,* or Medicare Plan D and supplemental policies reflect the current date. Know the name of your Medicare supplemental health and Plan D insurance carrier(s) such as Blue Cross/Blue Shield, Humana or Mutual of Omaha.

- *Automobile insurance.* Although you take the train or plane into the city you're visiting, you may rent or borrow a car when you arrive. You must have a current driver's license and confirmation of your current auto insurance coverage.

- Leave a *photocopy of these documents* (insurance policies, driver's license, social security card) with a relative, close friend or your lawyer in the event you lose the copy you're carrying with you. Make certain the person you choose can phone or forward this information quickly (overnight mail, fax or email), if necessary.

- *Medicare Rights Center.* Contact the Medicare Rights Center if you are a Senior Citizen. This consumer group can be reached at 1-800-333-4114, or at their Web site www.medicarerights.org.
Before you complete your travel plans, you will want to ask them about any exclusions or conditions that are not covered under your plans. For example, your Medicare plan *may not* cover your medical needs outside the United States.

- *Medical evacuation insurance.* Travelers with disabilities venturing into remote areas of the country (or outside the United States) should be aware of Medical Evacuation Insurance that offers emergency air evacuation to medical facilities. Evacuation Insurance also may be offered through your employer, or through your general health insurance policies. Several companies offering this insurance can be found listed on the Internet. Know the parameters of their policies before you subscribe. Travel agents also may be knowledgeable about the details of this insurance.

- *Prescription refills.* Do not expect your physician to remember the names of your medications, your prescription numbers or other pertinent medical data. Although some clinics store medical prescriptions and other medical information on a system wide computer, other medical clinics store their medical files in a central office, requiring that your physician request your records. Transferring these files can take at least two or three days. Ask your physician about his/her system.

Personal Experience

SMA—When I visited my daughter, I carefully counted the number of pills I would need, taking along several extra of each prescription. Unexpectedly, I extended my visit and found myself short in each prescription. Fortunately, I found the national pharmacy I had been using at home a few miles from my daughter's home. The pharmacy in Tennessee contacted my Minneapolis pharmacy that kept the original prescription on file. I picked up my refill the following morning and enjoyed my extended visit. Target, Walgreen and other pharmacies offer this convenience. Before you leave home ask your pharmacy whether they also offer a similar service.

Carry-on and Checked Baggage

Decide which bag(s) you will check and which you will carry-on. Since rules change, contact your carrier about the number of bags allowed, as well as weight and size limitations.

Carry-on bags

Airlines have restricted the use of carry-on bags and carry-on items such as toothpaste, lipstick gels, Vaseline and other liquid and gel products. The liquids and gels must be in a 3-ounce or less container (tube, jar, etc.) and placed in a 1-quart sealable clear plastic bag. Presently, airlines allow each passenger one sealable bag. Medicines in sealable bags do not count. Coffee or other beverages must be purchased in the terminal once you have cleared security. You may then take them with you on the plane. Trains and buses currently allow a briefcase, a small piece of luggage (that fits under the seat or in the overhead), and a purse or personal item as carry-on items. However, this varies from carrier to carrier, so ask your travel agent, Amtrak, Greyhound or your specific carrier.

Personal Experience

SMA—An inexpensive packing technique I have used for years requires only a few clear plastic bags (zip lock preferred) ranging in capacity from a sandwich bag to a gallon size. The Transportation Security Administration now requires the quart size plastic bag for packing containers of liquid and gels.

T-shirts, swimsuits, and lingerie, for example, can be placed together (i.e., lingerie with lingerie, t-shirts with t-shirts, etc.) and tucked into your baggage. These see-through bags allow a quick inspection if security guards open your bag. You can help prevent both carry-on and checked bags from being left in disarray after inspectors have looked through your baggage.

Tips for diabetics
Carry a small cooler for insulin pens or vials of insulin that require refrigeration, if you travel by bus, car, plane or train. This will depend on the length of your trip. Check online with The American Diabetes Association at www.childrenwithdiabetes.com or www.diabetes.org or contact your physician or pharmacist for availability of coolers.

Guard your Security

Gather together all the items you are taking onboard before you enter the line for a security check. If you travel by plane, you, and all your carry-on items will be screened, along with your wheelchair, service animal and/or other assistive devices. Rail lines and bus lines will require identification. Amtrak has refused to check my luggage without government picture ID (driver's license, for example).

If you are asked to remove clothing during the security screening process, and feel embarrassed or uncomfortable, request a private screening. All passengers have the right to a private screening.

Inform the security guards if you have a cochlear implant in your ear and show them a medical card from your physician.

Travel and Food

Passengers whose health requires food at specific intervals (i.e., every four hours, at noon, etc.) should bring food for snacks and meals. Airport security now requires that you purchase drinks, such as coffee, within the terminal *after* you pass through the security check point. Train terminals frequently do not have restaurants on the premises, but most long distance trains have food in their dining or club cars. Select suitable snacks such as fruit, peanut butter and crackers, candy or a bag lunch in the event weather or an emergency causes a travel delay.

> *Personal Experience*
>
> *SMA—During a holiday trip by rail, our train lost power in the food service area for over an hour. Their microwave cooking units, toaster and other electrical appliances were not available to provide hot food. The Dining Car was able to extend the lunch hour to make-up for the lost time during the regularly scheduled lunchtime, but then closed for dinner. The Club Car offered cold sandwiches, chips and other snack food. We highly suggest you take a back-up source of food for these unexpected occasions. Candy or orange juice can help boost blood sugar levels of passengers with diabetes.*

We review for you the general food policies followed by each of the public transportation lines. These may change from time to time, but these are based on our current information.

Airlines
Ask whether meals, snacks or refreshments will be served during your trip and whether they charge a fee. Many airlines no longer offer complimentary meals, but may allow you the option of purchasing a meal or snack onboard. Other airlines may offer you a can of soda or juice, a cookie or a bag of pretzels.

Amtrak.
Food is available for purchase in the Club car and Dining car on certain trains. First class passengers are given complimentary meal tickets for use in the dining car. Some rail lines may leave a basket of snacks in your private compartment or bedroom. Persons with disabilities can request that an attendant serve their food at their seat or in their compartment or bedroom.

Automobile.
Some travelers need to time their meals carefully to meet their special dietary needs. Carry a road map and take note of specific restaurants along the route. Road signs also offer helpful information. For example, you may need to ignore restaurants known for their luscious pies, ice cream and other desserts and stop for the salad bar and roasted chicken or turkey. Food choices can affect your health.

Greyhound.
Greyhound and some long distance buses such as Megabus stop along the route. Greyhound usually schedules stops at their Greyhound Restaurants, giving passengers the opportunity to purchase food and magazines. We suggest you bring along snacks or pick-up fresh fruit or candy if you need something to boost your blood sugar.

A Little Extra Assist

Traveling with assistive devices requires planning and knowing how and where your carrier allocates storage areas.

Personal Experiences

SMA & BR—A friend told us she always put her powered wheelchair in the cargo area of the plane where the rest of the checked baggage is stored. But, she cautioned that she takes it directly to the plane herself. At the gate she makes sure a door tag is attached with the destination written clearly on the tag. Then she says she checks to make certain the chair tag is marked with the same place she is going! She recalls her two worst-case scenarios.

"Twice my chair was left on the jet way, so I always make a point, once I get on the plane, to remind the attendants to make certain THAT chair is put on THIS plane!"

If you have visual limitations, pack a folding white cane, even though you do not use one at home. Place your folding white cane in your briefcase or a large purse under the seat or in the overhead bin. In cities and other heavily populated areas your cane acts as a signal to others that you may need extra space or more time as you move from place to place.

Airlines
Stow rigid canes and crutches in the cargo area or in the cabin's closet. Security rules will require that you stow these assistive devices out of your reach. Security guards and sky marshals are aware that crutches and canes can be used as weapons and take these measures to protect all passengers.

Personal Experience

SMA: I noticed a sticker in one of the cabs in Chicago indicating that persons with wheelchairs were welcome in that cab. When I inquired about the service, the driver told me most cabs in Chicago offer the same assistance.

Most airports, bus stations and staffed train stations make wheelchairs available for passengers with disabilities who are boarding or arriving at the terminal. (See chapters on plane, train and bus travel.) Consider taking your own if you cannot confirm rental availability and will rely on a wheelchair at your destination.

Travel with your powered wheelchair
If you are traveling with a powered wheelchair, the carrier will ask you to check-in early. You also will need patience as you go through the steps necessary to stow your wheelchair in the plane's cargo bin. Ask train and bus reservation agents about their policy for taking wheelchairs onboard.

Personal Experiences

SMA & BR: Another friend, who travels frequently, suggests that wheelchair users ask that the airline attach a "door tag" to their chair. This helps ensure your chair is delivered to the door of the plane when you deplane. You also can avoid transferring into an airline chair at the door of the plane, instead transferring directly into your own wheelchair for the ride to baggage claim. You also can remain in your own chair, avoiding a second transfer at baggage claim. Ask for a "door tag" at the gate when you check-in. Tags are usually available, but do ask.

Handling Wheelchair Batteries

The battery on your wheelchair will be treated separately from the wheelchair, depending on the type battery you use.

Spillable wet cell batteries

Sulfuric acid can, if spilled, corrode your wheelchair's wiring, the wheelchair, and parts of the aircraft. Most airlines refuse to carry a spillable battery unless it is removed and stored in a chemical-proof, spill-proof container. If the carrier removes the battery from the wheelchair because of the DOT hazardous waste regulations, the carrier must provide packaging that meets safety requirements. Wheelchair batteries are packaged with no fee to the passenger.

Non-spillable dry cell, gel-cell batteries

Since 1995, nonspillable dry cell (gel-cell) batteries must be marked and identified as nonspillable, according to

DOT rules. In addition, DOT hazardous materials regulations provide that it is unnecessary to remove a battery marked as nonspillable. If a battery is *not marked* as nonspillable, it can be removed from the wheelchair. During the loading and storing process, the battery must always be in an upright position.

Do not drain the battery
A wheelchair battery may not be drained.

Packaging a disconnected battery
If DOT regulations require disconnecting the battery (because it contains hazardous materials); you can request packaging for the battery that meets safety requirements. The carrier cannot charge you for such packaging. Make certain you ship your battery charger with you.

Assistive devices require extra attention, extra care, and extra time when you are traveling. As with all traveling, planning ahead helps your trip go smoothly. Listen to the words of one of our friends:

Personal Experience

SMA: A friend of years past, who became a wheelchair user following a spinal cord injury told me, "I've found I can do most things anyone else does. It just takes me a little longer." His sense of self-confidence was apparent as he described boarding a plane with his wheelchair.

May You Have a Healthy and Happy Voyage!

CHAPTER 9

LET THE JOURNEY BEGIN

We began this book with a description of two journeys. Both were marked by difficulties and stumbling blocks. Both were also marked by happy endings. Our experience shows us that most of us return from our travels full of happy memories and eager to plan our next adventure. When this happens, we encourage you to share with others what you did to plan for that successful trip. Become a mentor for other people with disabilities who have not yet dared to expand their travel horizons.

If on the other hand you encountered difficulties of any kind, we urge you to sort out what happened and why, so that in the future you can eliminate the rough patches. If your airline, bus, or train company failed to live up to your expectations, or if you were denied your rights as a passenger with a disability, address the problem quickly and succinctly. Write or call the airline or other provider. State clearly what happened, how it affected your safety and enjoyment, and what recompense you expect as a result of these unnecessary inconveniences. Don't be shy about what you ask for. Be persistent until you receive what you believe you deserve.

All of us who are disabled have both rights and responsibilities as we travel. Being a strong advocate on our own behalf (and on behalf of those who will follow in our tracks) is part of that package. I have a button I am very fond of which reads, "If you accept what they give you, you deserve what you get." Our friend Jim who developed pulmonary edema was not told that he had to request medical oxygen several hours before the flight. The young mother who climbed the steps to the plane carrying a stroller and her child with a disability was unaware that she was entitled to assistance from airline personnel. Familiarity with the rights and responsibilities of travelers with disabilities could have avoided these stresses.

Take responsibility for planning ahead and for being knowledgeable of policies and rules. We hope the resources and reference material which follows (beginning on page 105) will expedite your planning and heighten the enjoyment of your travel. At the time of publication, all were current. Changes in travel resources and regulations occur, so check to see that they are current and still work for you.

Best of luck with your travel. May it open to you new worlds, and may it enhance your confidence in yourself as it provides you with new freedom and new frontiers.

BON VOYAGE!

Endnotes

Chapter 1

For futher information, see Endnotes for Chapter 2.

Chapter 2

1 Air Carrier Access Act (ACAA): United States of America, Department of Transportation, Office of Aviation Enforcement and Proceedings Washington, DC; 14 CFR Part 382, Nondiscrimination on the Basis of Disability in Air Travel. (See also References and Resources section.)

2 *New Horizons* can be downloaded at the website: www.dot.gov or, more directly, at www.dotcr.ost.dot.gov (See also References and Resources section.)

3 The U.S. Department of Transportation (DOT), in their publication *New Horizons: Information for the Air Traveler with a Disability*, states even though "… this disability may offend, annoy, or be an inconvenience to crew-members or other passengers."

Chapter 3

1 If attendants choose to provide you with an individual briefing, the DOT handbook, *New Horizons,* notes that an individual briefing " . . .must be done inconspicuously and as discretely as possible," (p. 7). You cannot be quizzed about the briefing material.

2 Transportation Security Administration, U.S. Department of Homeland Security.

References and Resources

Please Note: Both the websites and telephone numbers listed below are subject to change without notice. We urge readers to search the internet for current information and updates.

Access Board, Independent Federal Agency
1331 F Street, NW
Ste 1000
Washington, DC 20004-1111
1-800-872-2253
1-800-993-2822
www.access-board.gov

Air Carrier Access Act
Hotline: 1-800-778-4838
File Complaints: 1-800-775-2235
TTY: 1-800-455-9880
(See also US Department of Transportation Civil Rights for internet access.)

American Diabetes Association
www.diabetes.org

Amtrak (US Rail Service)
www.amtrak.com
Send complaints in writing to:
   Amtrak Customer Relations
   60 Massachusetts Ave NE
   Washington, DC 20002

Aviation Consumer Protection
Air Consumer Protection Div
US Department of Transportation (DOT)
400 7th Street, SW
Washington, DC 20590
www.airconsumer@dot.ost.gov
Download or print complaint forms
   Email: airconsumer@dot.gov

Centers for Independent Living
www.virtualcil.net/cil
See map at web site for each state.

Federal Aviation Administration (FAA)
www.faa.gov
Provides airport status for delays, weather, tips for safe travel

Federal Motor Carrier Safety Administration (FMCSA)
Insurance: 1-202-358-7000
Safety Rating: 1-703-280-4001
www.fmcsa.dot.gov

Gimp-on-the-Go
www.gimponthego.com
Online publication for persons with disabilities.

Medicare Rights Center
www.medicarerights.org
1-800-333-4114

Paratransit Services, Inc.
4810 Auto Center Way, Ste Z
Bremerton, WA 98312
1-360-377-7176
www.paratransit.net

Transportation Security Administration
www.tsa.gov
Tips on security rules, items not permitted to be carried on planes, and more

US Department of Transportation (DOT)
www.dot.gov
Provides information for automobile, motor coach, rail and plane safety.

US Department of Transportation Civil Rights (DOTCR)
www.dotcr.ost.dot.gov
Read or download and print the *New Horizons: Information for the Air Traveler with a Disability*
Go to: www.dotcr.ost.dot.gov and enter New Horizons in the SEARCH window in the upper left-hand corner of the home page.

NOTES

Major Domestic (US) Airlines

Please Note: Both the websites and telephone numbers listed below are subject to change without notice. We urge readers to search the internet for current information and updates.

	Telephone	TDD/TTY
AirTran Airways www.airtran.com	1-800-247-8726	
Alaska Airlines www.alaskaairlines.com	1-800-252-7522	1-800-682-2221
American Airlines www.aa.com	1-800-223-5436	1-800-543-1586
America West (See: USAirways)		
Continental Airlines www.continental.com	1-800-523-3273	1-800-343-9195
Delta Airlines www.delta.com	1-800-221-1212	1-800-831-4488
Frontier www.frontierairlines.com	1-800-432-1359	

Major Domestic (US) Airlines cont'd

	Telephone	TDD/TTY
Jet Blue www.jetblue.com	1-800-538-2583	
Midwest Airline www.midwestairlines.com	1-800-452-2022	1-800-872-3608
Northwest Airlines www.nwa.com	1-800-225-2525	1-800-328-2298
Southwest Airlines www.southwest.com	1-800-435-9792	1-800-533-1305
Sun Country Airlines www.suncountry.com	1-800-359-6786	
Ted Airlines www.flyted.com	1-800-225-5833	1-800-323-0170
United Airlines www.united.com	1-800-864-8331	1-800-323-0170
USAirways www.usairways.com	1-800-428-4322	

Major Domestic Airport Codes

City	Code	City	Code
Atlanta	ATL	Newark	EWR
Baltimore	BWI	New Orleans	MSY
Birmingham	BHM	New York JFK	JFK
Boston	BOS	New York LGA	LGA
Burbank	BUR	Oakland, CA	OAK
Charlotte	CLT	Ontario, CA	ONT
Chicago Midway	MDW	Orange Co. CA	SNA
Chicago O'Hare	ORD	Orlando	MCO
Cincinnati	CVG	Philadelphia	PHL
Cleveland	CLE	Phoenix	PHX
Dallas Fort Worth	DFW	Pittsburgh	PIT
Dallas Love Field	DAL	Portland	PDX
Denver	DEN	Raleigh/Durham	RDU
Detroit	DTW	Reno	RNO
Fort Lauderdale	FLL	Sacramento	SMF
Honolulu	HNL	Salt Lake City	SLC
Houston Hob	HOU	San Antonio	SAT
Houston Int	IAH	San Diego	SAN
Indianapolis	IND	San Francisco	SFO
Kansas City	MCI	San Jose	SJC
Las Vegas	LAS	Seattle	SEA
Los Angeles	LAX	St. Louis	STL
Memphis	MEM	Tampa	TPA
Miami, FL	MIA	Wash. DC Dulles	IAD
Minneapolis	MSP	Wash. DC National	DCA
Nashville	BNA		

This is not a complete list of US airports, but provides the reader with some of the largest airports in the USA.

CHECKLIST FOR PACKING

Include these items as needed.

Personal Identification

- ☐ Driver's license (current)
- ☐ Luggage Tags (outside and inside luggage)
- ☐ Non-driver's identification, if needed (current)
- ☐ Insurance identification cards
- ☐ Tickets (correct date, carrier, destination, etc)

Prescription for healthy travel

- ☐ Explanation of your medical condition, signed by your doctor. (This is especially important if you use a syringe and needle as part of your medical treatment.)
- ☐ Prescription medicines (amount you will need plus enough for 2-3 extra days)
- ☐ Copies of your prescription(s)
- ☐ Non-prescription medication(s)
- ☐ Personal physician's name, office address and phone number
- ☐ Personal pharmacy's/pharmacist's name and phone number
- ☐ Small cooler for insulin pens

CHECKLIST FOR PACKING FOR TRIP

The following are supplies and devices you may want to include for your trip as needed.

- ☐ Binoculars (travel size) for low vision and for viewing items at a distance
- ☐ Eyeglasses and Contact Lens supplies (cleaning agents, etc)
- ☐ Insect repellant, as appropriate
- ☐ Liquid for cleansing contact lens for eyeglasses
- ☐ Magnifying device/small light for reading
- ☐ Prescription for replacement eyeglass lens or contacts
- ☐ Sun glasses
- ☐ Sunscreen
- ☐ White collapsible cane, as needed
- ☐ Hearing aids and supplies
- ☐ Extra hearing-aid batteries
- ☐ Dry-aid kits to help eliminate moisture in your hearing aids (this can improve the performace of your hearing aid and should be used regularly)
- ☐ Extra batteries for flash lights, hearing aids, and other electronic devices.

MY LIST OF ITEMS TO PACK

PACKED	TO PICK UP BEFORE TRIP						

MY LIST OF ITEMS TO PACK

PACKED	TO PICK UP BEFORE TRIP

Sue Maris Allen, MPH, MSW

In 1999 I experienced two strokes that left me with partial paralysis of the right side of my body and impaired vision in my left eye.

I am a nurse by profession, receiving my Bachelor's degree in Public Health Nursing, and a double Masters in Public Health and Social Work from the University of Minnesota. Applying the expertise of a persistent team of physicians and physical therapists, as well as my own medical knowledge, we charted my course of rehabilitation with the goal of resuming my favorite activities, including travel.

For inspiration in this challenging process, I recalled the indomitable spirits of two of my closest relatives. By her ninetieth year, my great Grandma B had been a survivor of multiple strokes but played games with me, told me stories and was a wonderful, active part of my toddler life. My father, too, became a wheelchair user resulting from a farm equipment accident during his last year of life. He refused to allow his disability to interfere with his interest and involvement in farm and home activities, especially in the lives of his four young daughters. My family's tradition never permitted a physical limitation to impact their enjoyment of family, life and work.

The extent of my recovery could be deemed extraordinary. I regained most of my mobility. I did, however, have some permanent residual effects of the strokes that continue with me to this day: I walk more slowly and cautiously than I once did, and do not always see things if they are in my lower left field of vision.

Eventually the first opportunity arose for me to travel alone, flying to Arizona for a family celebration. Considering the positive response from the airline agent who made my reservations, I expected this flight to be no different than the many previous flights I had made in my life.

However, I had an unexpected awakening. Cabin and gate attendants greeted my requests for help (already noted in their computers) by sending me to wait at the end of the line. I felt surprise and dismay at the negative impact their attitude had on my feelings of comfort and confidence as a traveler. I had considered these changes in my physical abilities to be comparatively small. But, my need for a little more help or attention was met with impatience, or worse, disrespect.

Disillusioned, I shared my experiences with my friend Barbara, who has been blind for 40 years. She related similar experiences, and gave me some positive tips for future travel. I felt better, having the support of a more experienced traveler with a disability. I knew I was not alone.

Frequent legal discussions among the three lawyers in my family aroused my curiosity. What rights were available to me, a traveler with a disability? I began to study laws such as the Air Carrier Access Act. I realized that there were laws and rights that could be enforced to ensure that I was a respected valued traveler.

After advising many friends and relatives on these issues, Barbara and I decided to combine our resources and create the book Wheeling and Dealing.

Today I live in Minneapolis, Minnesota with my husband Richard who is semi-retired from the practice of law. I enjoy traveling as much as I did before my strokes. In the past year alone, I have traveled by plane, train, bus, and automobile to visit our children in California, Illinois, and Tennessee.

Today travelers with disabilities enjoy travel, not only as a luxury, but as a well-protected right. My hope is that the many stories, laws, and facts in this book will empower anyone with a disability to embrace their right to travel, armed with knowledge and confidence.

The Reverend Barbara Ramnaraine, B.A.

Four or five years ago, my friend Sue and I began thinking about writing this book. We are both people with disabilities, we had both had bad experiences while traveling, and we had both become good advocates on our own behalf. While we believed that the book would take us four or five months, as you can see, we were wrong.

I was born in 1934, the oldest of three children. My parents were both doctors, though my mother never practiced after my birth. By the time I was eighteen months old, it was evident that I had limited vision. I had very thick glasses and even with them, I almost put my nose on whatever I wanted to see. I knew very early that I could not see like other kids. Thanks to my parents treating me just like any other child, however, I didn't know that I was disabled until I was an adult.

The Minneapolis school system had wonderful special-education classes. We were mainstreamed before that word was invented some thirty years later. The only thing that I didn't do in school was to play basketball and other sorts of ball games. The physical education teacher made me jump rope instead, and I hated being different.

Even in elementary school, I was fond of writing. This interest grew with the passing years. In high school, I was the editor of the editorial page for the school newspaper. By college I thought I wanted to be a journalist. I took creative writing and the first course in journalism my freshman year.

Then chemistry came along, and I forgot all abut journalism or creative writing. I graduated with a minor in education and a major in chemistry.

I married, had my first child, and taught in small schools in South Dakota and western Minnesota the first three years after graduating from college.

After that, for the next 25 years, I devoted myself to raising my three children. Writing was not lost, but it certainly was not on the front burner either.

In 1984, I embarked on an entirely new career. By that time, the little vision I had as a child and young adult had been lost. I was left with only a bit of light perception. I was ordained an Episcopal deacon on January 25, 1984. From that time on, sermons proved to be my primary writing. About the same time, I was invited to become a member of The Presiding Bishop's Task Force on Accessibility. This was a group which set the course for disability ministry for the Episcopal Church nationally.

I have cherished the 23 plus years of my diaconal ministry and even more, being a part of making the church aware of the gifts and needs of people with disabilities. There has been enormous progress made in welcoming people with disabilities into the full life of the church. However, there is much more to be done, and I am glad that I am still a part of making that happen.

INDEX

A

ACAA. See Air Carrier Access Act (1986)

Access Board, Independent Federal Agency, 105

accessible Amtrak stations, 46-47

accessible equipment, Amtrak, 50-51; Greyhound, 62

accessible passenger cars (Amtrak), available equipment in, 50-51; bedrooms, 50, 52; Club Cars, 52; overview, 49-50; reserving accessible space, 51-52

advance notice rule, for air travel, 13-14

Air Carrier Access Act (1986), advance notice rule, 13-14; assistance rule, 9-10; contact information for, 105; exit rows rule, 11-12; future changes in rules, 18-19; group travel rule, 14-15; overview, 9, 103; Personal Care Attendant (PCA) rule, 15-16; reporting violations of, 17-18; rules of, 9-18; seating rule, 10-11; service animals rule, 16; travel information, 16-17; unattended passengers rule, 13

airline contact information (domestic), 109-110

airport codes, 23-24, 111

AirTran Airways contact information, 109

air travel, advance notice requirement for, 13-14; air miles, 42-43; airport/city codes, 23-24, 111; arrival procedures, 37-38; arrival time, 6; assistive devices, 40-41, 97; baggage, 24, 27-28, 83, 92-93; beverage service, 28, 42, 92, 94; boarding airplanes, 6-7, 23; booking, 21-22; check-in, 27-28; confirming reservations, 23; connecting flights, 25-27; direct flights, 24-25; domestic airline contact information, 109-110; e-tickets, 22-23; exit rows, 11-12; flight selection, 24-27; food service, 35-36, 95; getting assistance with, 9-10; group travel, 14-15; hard-of-hearing passengers, 33; humor, sense of, 34; kiosks, 22-23. 42; medical oxygen, 34-35; motorized wheelchairs/scooters, 38-40, 97-98; overview, 21; Personal Care Attendant (PCA), 15-16; preboarding, 7; prohibited items, 41-42; proposed changes, 41-43; safety briefings, 33-34; seating, 10-11; security, 29-33, 41-42; service animals, 16, 32-33; tips for, 5-7, 21-41; unattended passengers, 13; wheelchair requests, 28-29

Alaska Airlines contact information, 109

Allen, Sue Maris, personal story, 3-5, 117-118

American Airlines contact information, 109

American Diabetes Association Web site, 93, 105

America West contact information, 109

Amtrak, accessible passenger cars, 49-52; accessible stations, 46-47; baggage, 52-53, 83; beverage service, 52; contact information, 46, 47, 51, 55, 57, 105; discounts for, 53; Fast-Trak machine, 49; food service, 52, 54-55, 95; medical oxygen, 56; overview, 45-46; purchasing tickets for, 47-49; security rules, 55-56; service animals, 54; smoking on, 54; Web site, 49, 57, 105

arrival procedures, air travel, 37-38

arrival time, air travel, 6, 25-26; Greyhound, 63; overview, 81-82

assistive devices, air travel, 40-41, 97; Greyhound, 63-64; overview, 96-97

Aviation Consumer Protection contact information, 106

B

baggage, air travel, 24, 27-28, 83, 92-93; Amtrak, 52-53, 83; Greyhound, 60, 64-65, 83; overview, 92-93; size and weight limitations of, 83-84

batteries for motorized wheelchairs/scooters, 39-40, 98-99

beverages, air travel, 28, 42, 92, 94; Amtrak, 52; proposed changes for air travel, 42

boarding, airplanes, 6-7, 23; Amtrak, 49; Greyhound, 63; preboarding, 7

boarding pass. See boarding

booking, See also ticketing: air travel, 21-22; Amtrak, 47-49; Greyhound, 60-61

books, packing, 85-86

bus travel. See charter bus travel; Greyhound

C

carry-on baggage, air travel, 27-28, 92; Amtrak, 52-53; Greyhound, 60, 64-65

car travel, "access guides," 78; being your own advocate, 79-80; Centers for Independent Living, 77-78; food service, 95; insulin users, 79; Internet research for, 77-78; licensing, 77; overview, 77

Centers for Independent Living Web site, 106

charter bus travel, See also Greyhound: company information, 73; driver information, 73; insurance, 74; overview, 71-72; references, 74; safety rating, 74; special needs travelers, 74-75; subcontracting agreements, 75-76; vehicle standards, 72-73

checked baggage, air travel, 24, 83, 92-93; Amtrak, 52-53; Greyhound, 64-65

check-in, air travel, 27-28; Greyhound, 63
checklists, packing, 113-116
city codes, 23-24, 111
cochlear implants, air travel with, 30-31
complaints, air travel, 17-18; Complaints Resolution Official (CRO), 17; Greyhound, 69
confirming reservations, for air travel, 23
connecting flights, 25-27
Continental Airlines contact information, 109
curbside check-in, 27-28

D

defibrillator, air travel with, 30; precautions, 88
Delta Airlines contact information, 109
Department of Transportation (DOT), Civil Rights (DOTCR) Web site, 107; contact information, 74; "New Horizons: Information for the Air Traveler with a Disability," 9, 103; violations hotline, 17; Web site, 7, 107
diabetics, travel tips for, 93
direct flights, 24-25
discount fares, air travel, 25; Amtrak, 53; Greyhound, 61, 66
disputes, air travel, 17-18
documents, insurance, 89-91; medical, 88-89; personal identification, 87
DOT. See Department of Transportation (DOT)

E

electronic devices, 87-88
e-tickets, for air travel, 22-23
exit rows, air travel, 11-12

F

FAA. See Federal Aviation Administration (FAA)
Fast-Trak machine (Amtrak), 49
Federal Aviation Administration (FAA) Web site, 7, 43, 106
Federal Motor Carrier Safety Administration (FMCSA), 72, 74, 106
flight selection, connecting flights, 25-27; direct flights, 24-25

FMCSA. See Federal Motor Carrier Safety Administration (FMCSA)

food service, air travel, 35-36, 95; Amtrak, 48, 52, 54-55, 95; car travel, 95; Greyhound, 69, 96; overview, 94-95; proposed changes for air travel, 42

frequent flyer miles, 42-43

Frontier airline contact information, 109

G

Gimp-on-the-Go Web site, 33, 106

Greyhound, See also charter bus travel: accessible equipment, 62; arrival time, 63; assistive devices, 63-64; baggage, 60, 64-65, 83; boarding, 63; check-in, 63; contact information, 61, 67, 69; Disabilities Assist Line, 62; filing complaints, 69; food service, 69, 96; guidelines for traveling on, 63-68; medical information, 65; medical oxygen, 65; overview, 59-60; Personal Care Attendant (PCA), 66-68; personal identification, 66; priority seating, 66; prohibited items, 65; proof-of-disability, 66; reservations, 60; service animals, 68; smoking, 66; ticketing, 60-61; travel with minors, 68; Web site, 67

group air travel, 14-15

H

hard-of-hearing passengers, air travel for, 33

I

identification, air travel, 28; checklist, 113; documents, 87; Greyhound, 63, 66

implanted devices (surgically), air travel with, 30

insurance, charter bus travel, 74; documents, 89-91; medical evacuation, 90-91

J

Jet Blue contact information, 110

K

kiosks, air travel boarding passes, 22-23; mailing banned items, 42

M

medical documents, checklist for, 113; Greyhound, 65; importance of carrying, 88; what to carry, 88-89

medical equipment, 86

medical evacuation insurance, 90-91

medical insurance cards, 89

medical oxygen, air travel with, 34-35; Amtrak, 56; Greyhound, 65

Medicare Rights Center, 90, 106

medications, importance of carrying, 88-89; overview, 86

Midwest Airlines contact information, 110

minors, traveling on Greyhound with, 68

motorized wheelchairs/scooters, air travel with, 97-98; batteries for, 39-40, 98-99; overview, 38-39

N

National Library Service for the Blind and Physically Handicapped, 85-86

"New Horizons: Information for the Air Traveler with a Disability" (DOT), 9, 103

Northwest Airlines contact information, 110

O

oxygen, air travel with, 34-35; Amtrak, 56; Greyhound, 65

P

pacemaker, air travel with, 30; precautions, 88

packing, baggage, 83-84; books, 85-86; checklist, 113-116; coat/jacket, 85; overview, 82-83; shoes, 84-85

paper tickets, for air travel, 22

Paratransit Services, Inc. Web site, 107

passengers (air travel), rule for leaving unattended, 13

Personal Care Attendant (PCA), air travel with, 15-16; Greyhound, 66-67

personal identification. See identification

preboarding, See also boarding: air travel, 7

prohibited items, air travel, 27, 41-42; Greyhound, 65; proposed changes for air travel, 41

proof-of-disability (Greyhound), 66
proposed changes in air travel, 41-43
purchasing tickets. See ticketing

R

Ramnaraine, Barbara, personal story, 1-3, 119-120
references, for charter bus travel, 74
requesting wheelchairs, 28-29
reservations, air travel, 13-14, 23, 43; Amtrak, 47-49, 51; Greyhound, 60

S

safety briefings, air travel, 33-34
safety rating, for charter bus travel, 74
scooters. See motorized wheelchairs/scooters
seating, air travel, 10-12; Amtrak, 47-49, 51-52; Greyhound, 66
security, See also security (airport)
security (airport), cochlear implants, 30-31; overview, 29-30, 93-94; pacemaker/defibrillator, 30; proposed changes for, 41-42; "secured" area, 31-32; service animals, 32-33; shoes, 32; surgically implanted devices, 30
security, Amtrak, 52, 55-56; Greyhound, 66
sense of humor, 34
service animals, air travel with, 16, 32-33; Amtrak, 54; Greyhound, 68
shoes, air travel, 32; packing, 84-85
smoking, Amtrak, 54; Greyhound, 66
snacks. See food service
Southwest Airlines contact information, 110
subcontracting agreements, charter bus travel, 75-76
Sun Country Airlines contact information, 110
supplies checklist, 113

T

Ted Airlines contact information, 110
3-1-1 icon for allowable security items, 27
ticket counter check-in (air travel), 27-28

ticketing, See also booking: airline e-tickets, 22-23; Amtrak, 47-49; Greyhound, 60-61

tips, for air travel, 5-7; for diabetics, 93

train travel. See Amtrak

Transportation, Department of. See Department of Transportation (DOT)

Transportation Security Administration (TSA), 3-1-1 icon, 27; Web site, 7, 41, 43, 83, 107

travel information, providing during air travel, 16-17

U

United Airlines contact information, 110

USAirways contact information, 110

W

Web sites, Access Board, Independent Federal Agency, 105; American Diabetes Association, 93, 105; Amtrak, 49, 57, 105; Aviation Consumer Protection, 106; Centers for Independent Living, 106; Children with Diabetes, 93; Department of Transportation (DOT), 7, 107; Department of Transportation Civil Rights (DOTCR), 107; Federal Aviation Administration (FAA), 7, 43, 106; Federal Motor Carrier Safety Administration (FMCSA), 106; Gimp-on-the-Go, 33, 106; Greyhound, 67; major domestic airlines, 109-110; Medicare Rights Center, 90, 106; Paratransit Services, Inc., 107; Transportation Security Administration (TSA), 7, 41, 43, 83, 107

wheelchairs, batteries, 98-99; motorized, 38-40, 97-98; requests for, 28-29

Printed in the United States
123287LV00004B/1-99/P